Fetal

Electrocardiography

CARDIOPULMONARY MEDICINE FROM IMPERIAL COLLEGE PRESS

Series Editor: Robert H. Anderson
National Heart & Lung Institute, London

Published:

Controversies in the Description of Congenitally Malformed Hearts
(*with video*)
    R. H. Anderson

The Conduction System in the Mammalian Heart — An Anatomico-
histological Study of the Atrioventricular Bundle and the Purkinje Fibers
    S. Tawara; translated by K. Suma & M. Shimada

Fetal Electrocardiography
    E. M. Symonds, D. Sahota & A. Chang

Forthcoming:

Pulmonary Circulation: Basic Mechanisms to Clinical Practice
    J. M. B. Hughes & N. W. Morrell

Echocardiography in Congenital Heart Disease Made Simple
    S. Y. Ho, A. N. Redington, M. L. Rigby & R. H. Anderson

Fetal
Electrocardiography

E. Malcolm Symonds
University of Nottingham

Daljit Sahota
Allan Chang
The Chinese University of Hong Kong

Imperial College Press

Published by

Imperial College Press
57 Shelton Street
Covent Garden
London WC2H 9HE

Distributed by

World Scientific Publishing Co. Pte. Ltd.
P O Box 128, Farrer Road, Singapore 912805
USA office: Suite 1B, 1060 Main Street, River Edge, NJ 07661
UK office: 57 Shelton Street, Covent Garden, London WC2H 9HE

British Library Cataloguing-in-Publication Data
A catalogue record for this book is available from the British Library.

ISBN   1-86094-171-0

Printed in Singapore by Uto-Print

Contents

Introduction   ix
1. HISTORICAL DEVELOPMENT   1
  Early Observations   1
  Early Observations of the P & T Waves   4
  The P Wave and the QRS Complex   6
  Observations on the FECG Waveform in the 1970s
  with Appropriate Filtering   10
  New Methods of Signal Processing in the 1980s   12
  Clinical Trials and Observations in Recent Studies   14
  The QRS Complex   18
  Vectorcardiography   22
  Fetal Cardiac Arrythmias   23
  Tachyarrhythmias   24
  The Use of Abdominal Electrodes   25
  The R–R' Interval and Fetal Heart Rate   29
2. FETAL ADAPTATION   31
  What is Fetal Distress?   31
  Fetal Physiological Response to Hypoxia   33
   Intermediary metabolism   33
   Fetal blood gas and pH   34
   Cardiac response   35
  Cellular Effects of Hypoxia   36
   Oxygen radicals   36
   Membrane destruction   37
   DNA damage   38
   Cellular damage   38
   Adverse long-term outcome   38
  A Model for Fetal Distress   39

3. RESEARCH MODELS AND PREDICTION   41
   The Statistical Evaluation of Discrete Predictors   41
   The Statistical Evaluation of Continuous Predictors   43
   The Validation of Predictive Tests by Observational Studies   44
   The Validation of Predictive Tests by Clinical Trials   45
   The Inclusion of Both Intervention and Morbidity in
   a Clinical Trial of Predictive Tests   46
   The Hawthorne Effect   46
   Animal and Clinical Models of Study   47
4. THE ELECTRICAL SIGNAL, ITS ACQUISITION
   AND MEASUREMENT   49
   The Biophysics — How is the Fetal
   Electrocardiogram Produced?   49
   Acquisition of the Signal   53
     Obtaining the signal — Electrodes   53
     Non-penetrating electrodes   54
     Electrode characteristics   56
     Electrode–tissue interface   57
     Vectors   57
   Signal Detection and Enhancement   58
     Signal detection   58
     Enhancement   60
     Pitfalls of using time-coherent enhanced averaging   63
   Morphology and Time Measurement of the
   Enhanced Waveform   65
5. THE R-R′ INTERVAL AND THE CARDIOTOCOGRAPH   69
   Physiology of Fetal Heart Rate Regulation   69
   Regulation by the Autonomic Nervous System   70
   Regulation by Baroreceptors and Chemoreceptors   70
   Fetal Heart Rate Variability   71
   Short-Term Variability   71
   Long-Term Variability   72
   Fetal Behavioural States   73
   High Fetal Heart Rate Variability   73

Low Fetal Heart Rate Variability   73
Accelerations and Decelerations of the Fetal Heart Rate   74
  Accelerations   74
  Decelerations   75
  Early decelerations   75
  Late decelerations   76
  Variable decelerations   76
Interpretation of the CTG   77
Computerised Assessment of the RR Interval — New Definitions   78
  Baseline   79
  Baseline variability   79
  Accelerative episodes — accelerations   80
  Decelerative episodes — decelerations   80
Computerised Systems for the Interpretation of Antepartum
Fetal Heart Rate   81
Computerised Systems for the Interpretation of Intrapartum
Fetal Heart Rate   83
  Computerised estimation of baseline   83
  Computerised estimation of variability   84
  Computerised identification of decelerations   87
6. TIME INTERVALS AND MORPHOLOGY
  OF THE FETAL ECG   89
Analysis of the FECG   90
Development of an Analyser of the FECG   90
The PR Interval and the PR/FHR Relationship   92
P Wave Morphology and Area   92
The PR/FHR Relationship   93
The Application of PR/FHR to Clinical Trials   98
Prospective Trials   99
The QRS Complex   102
The R/S Ratio and Fetal Vector Cardiography   102
The QT Interval and the ST Segment   103
The T/QRS Ratio   104
7. FETAL CARDIAC ARRHYTHMIAS   108
Disorders of Cardiac Rhythms in the Fetus   108

Extrasystoles	109
Supraventricular Extrasystoles	110
Management	110
Escape Rhythms — The Bradycardias	111
Sinus Bradycardia	111
Management	111
Blocked Atrial Premature Beats	112
Complete Heart Block	112
Management	113
The Tachycardias	113
Supraventicular Tachycardias	113
Management	114
Atrial Flutter and Atrial Fibrillation	115
Management	116
Ventricular Tachycardia	116
8. INFORMATION INTERPRETATION AND TRANSFORMATION	117
The Transformation of Data	117
Simple transformations	117
Transformations based on theoretical assumptions	118
Serial transformations	120
Multivariate transformations	120
Neural networks	122
Organisation of the information	125
Object orientated structure of the data and algorithm	126
Presentation	129
Display of normality and abnormality	130
Vector display	130
9. CONCLUSIONS	132
Monitoring Methods Currently in Use	132
Problems with the Present Systems	135
Has the Fetal ECG Analysis Enhanced the Specificity of Fetal Monitoring?	136
The Way Forward	138
References	141

Introduction

There has been a number of excellent books published in recent years on the subject of fetal monitoring. Their primary function has been to examine the nature of the fetal heart rate and the physiology and pathophysiology of the regulation of the fetal heart beat and how this can be applied to the detection of fetal asphyxia and the prediction of adverse outcome for the fetus, either in terms of fetal death or brain damage. Over the last decade, there has been much debate and re-evaluation of the effectiveness of counting the fetal heart rate in achieving these objectives, although it must be pointed out that techniques of electronic monitoring were never actually introduced to prevent fetal damage but were introduced to prevent intrapartum fetal death. The initial historical studies produced very promising results in reducing intrapartum death rates as measured against the incidence of antepartum stillbirths. The Dublin randomised study of fetal heart rate monitoring (MacDonald *et al.*, 1985) was conducted on a large number of normal subjects and failed to show any difference in perinatal mortality between those infants monitored electronically and those monitored by intermittent auscultation. As fetal death in such a group has a very low prevalence, the study was inadequate to actually prove that point even though the numbers involved in the study were, by conventional standards, large.

The more difficult issue relates to the prevalence of cerebral palsy and whether electronic monitoring has had any impact on this problem. The widely held view is that the prevalence of cerebral palsy has, if anything, increased, although recent analysis of Bristol data (Pharoah, 1996) shows that the prevalence of cerebral palsy has fallen in mature infants but has risen in low birth weight infants, suggesting that the increased survival of very low birth weight infants has carried its own price and that intensive intrapartum observation of the fetus may have achieved its objectives as far as the mature fetus is concerned.

The fetus, as with the adult of the species, survives in a buffered environment and, therefore, its biochemical response to hypoxia and asphyxia is linear only until the extreme limits of compensation are reached. This is too late for intervention if the fetus is to be delivered in a healthy state. However, over-interpretation of abnormalities of the fetal heart rate has led to unnecessary intervention associated with high operative delivery rates.

Outcome measurements are further bedevilled by the knowledge that many infants who manifest cerebral palsy provide no evidence that the processes of parturition and fetal acidosis play any part in the pathology of the brain damage and where it must be concluded that either an episode of fetal asphyxia occurred before the onset of labour or that there was a genetic or infective problem that produced the abnormality.

This book is not about fetal monitoring although clearly it has implications for that subject. Over the past decade, the Departments of Obstetrics & Gynaecology at the University of Nottingham and the Chinese University of Hong Kong have collaborated on joint projects studying the nature of the fetal electrocardiogram waveform and intervals and its relationship to fetal health. The technical developments in Nottingham date back to the 1970s when the initial developments in signal acquisition and signal processing were produced in a collaboration between the Department of Obstetrics & Gynaecology and the Department of Electrical and Electronic Engineering.

The history of research on the fetal electrocardiogram dates back nearly a hundred years but progress has been intimately related to computer and chip technology. Unlike heart rate, the components of the ECG waveform are multiple and their interface is complex. The mass of information produced by detailed analysis of the ECG requires computer technology if the information is to be used in real time. Furthermore, the methods of analysis required to interpret the significance of the waveform pattern are numerous and complex. Understanding the fundamental physiology of electrical activity in the heart is a prerequisite for studying the subject of fetal electrocardiography. As we hope that this book will be a source of information and stimulation for both medical and engineering researchers in this field, we make no apologies for including basic descriptions of those subjects.

In assessing the relationship between the electrical activity in the fetal heart and in the conduction system, it is important to address the issues related to outcome and the biochemistry of fetal asphyxia. Increasingly, the research community has become aware of the fact that the relationship between fetal acidosis and outcome is complex. It is clear that some infants will survive profound fetal acidosis without suffering damage to the brain stem or cortical damage or intraventricular haemorrhage. The specific effect of reduced cerebral blood flow and the damage inflicted by free-oxygen radicals may be as important as any absolute changes in pH. The ability of the fetal heart to survive biochemical insults is considerable and the changes in the heart may therefore be at some remove from damage suffered by the brain. In using parameters from the fetal ECG as a tool for assessment of the health of the fetus, we are adopting a relatively oblique but accessible pathway.

In the interpretation of the parameters of the FECG, it is important to remember that ischaemia in the fetal myocardium has an entirely different pathogenesis to the common forms of ischaemic heart disease in the adult. The lesions that produce ischaemic heart disease are generally focal and occur in an intact individual. The fetus usually has normal coronary vessels but lives in an environment where it is entirely dependent on the placenta. In effect, it is permanently attached to a large dialysis unit. This means that the biochemical changes that occur during chronic asphyxia are generally mediated by the placenta but its capacity for coping with the different features induced by chronic oxygen deprivation may not be consistent. For example, asphyxia in either the fetus or the adult will produce a shift of K^+ from the intracellular location into the extracellular and intravascular spaces. As the placenta faces into a maternal circulation where the acid–base and electrolyte environment may be normal, does the fetus lose potassium into the maternal circulation, and if so, does the fetus effectively manifest a hypokalaemic intracellular environment? Ischaemic changes in the fetal heart are diffuse and therefore the changes in the ECG differ in many aspects from those seen in the adult.

With some notable exception, most of the attempts to use the fetal ECG for recognition of biochemical changes have followed the same pathway as the interpretation of heart rate and the R–R interval but the ECG offers many different measurements and therefore does not offer the constraints imposed by using a single parameter. Yet, most of the work in this field —

certainly until the 1980s — has tended to simply take single parameters and attempt to reproduce the same profile of analysis that has been used for heart rate. It is clear that the changes in the ECG are often subtle and will only become gross in the agonal stages of fetal asphyxia and are therefore of no value in preventing fetal demise. Furthermore, it is apparent that in using a single lead system attached to the presenting part of the fetus, there are constraints in measuring change in the morphology of the ECG. These difficulties are further compounded by the fact that any change of the position of the electrode may change the shape of the waveform, particularly in relation to the ST segment and T-wave configuration.

However, considerable advances have been made in the computerisation of data and in the techniques for removing electrical noise and artefacts by the use of sliding averages. Digitised data can be used not only in the continuous measurement of individual parameters and time intervals but also in examining the interaction between variables to see if the sensitivity and accuracy of fetal monitoring can be enhanced. Are we approaching the analysis of this mass of information in the right way or are there better techniques that would allow "computer" recognition of abnormal states? The application of neural networks takes a step in this direction, but so far, it has not been found to enhance precision. The method also has the disadvantage of being impossible to trace how a particular decision is reached. Provided that the end result allowed more efficient interpretation of the ECG, the use of such a technique would be justifiable, but that has so far not proven to be the case.

Whilst the primary objectives of this book are to review the history and the current status of fetal electrocardiography, we would be remiss if we did not take the opportunity to speculate on possible future technical developments in this field, and also to consider further the question of suitable outcome measurements and analysis of the ECG in relation to those factors.

Chapter 1

HISTORICAL DEVELOPMENT

Early Observations

Einthoven first described the use of a string galvanometer in 1901 to detect the presence of electrical activity in the adult heart and it was only five years later that Cremer (1906) first identified the fetal electrocardiogram from a combination of vaginal and abdominal electrodes. Cremer also used large oesophageal leads to obtain ECGs and in view of the discomfort that must have been involved for his volunteers and the crudity of the system of string galvanometry, it is quite remarkable that the original tracing, shown in Fig. 1.1, reported in his paper clearly shows a fetal QRS complex.

Interest in auscultation of the fetal heart developed in the 19th century with, amongst other observations, a book published by Kennedy in 1833 entitled *Observations of Obstetrical Auscultation* in which he observed that a slow return of the fetal heart rate (FHR) to its previous baseline following a deceleration was associated with "fetal sufferance" and that head

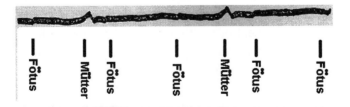

Fig. 1.1. The first recording of the fetal electrocardiogram in 1906 by Cremer using a string galvanometer (reprinted from Larks, 1959; copyright © Mosby, Inc.).

compression produced fetal bradycardia. Sixty years later, Winckel (1893) suggested that a FHR of less than 120 beats per minute (bpm) or greater than 160 bpm were indicative of fetal distress, so that by the beginning of the 20th century, the foundations of cardiotocography were already established. The potential difficulties and doubts were also noted when Seitz (1903) examined delayed decelerations in relation to fetal oxygenation and concluded that there was an overlap between physiological and pathological decelerations in predicting fetal hypoxia.

In view of the growing interest in fetal heart rate, perhaps it was surprising that over the next 24 years, only four papers appeared in the literature on the subject of the fetal electrocardiogram. Foa (1911), Haynal and Kellner (1923), and Maekawa and Toyoshima (1930) all used two external abdominal leads but the very low-voltage fetal signal and the high levels of background electrical artefacts made interpretation and evaluation of these signals difficult. It would have been much simpler to monitor the fetal heart beat by direct auscultation. Sach (1922) used abdomino-vaginal and abdomino-rectal leads in pregnant women to enhance the signal but the earlier success of Cremer was not repeated. It was clear that real advances would not occur until suitable advances could be made in amplification and filtering of the signal.

Maekawa and Toyoshima first employed a valve amplifier in their research in 1930 but the level of amplification was very limited before signal distortion occurred. The next publication appeared in 1938 when Bell, using abdominal electrodes, employed a balanced input amplifier to attenuate the electrical oscillation. Problems with baseline movement meant that the capacity of the condensers was reduced to 0.02 micro-farrad. Bell acknowledged that this technique removed the P&T waves which are of low frequency but clearly he did not consider that this was disadvantageous to the use and interpretation of the signal. Indeed, the prevailing use of the FECG to this day has remained the measurement of the time between successive R waves. In the same year, Strassman and Mussey produced a large study on 52 patients in late pregnancy. They recorded 70 electrocardiograms using abdominal electrodes and were able to detect a fetal electrocardiogram on 87% of the recordings with a failure to demonstrate any signal in 13% of the subjects.

The application of electrodes directly to aborted fetuses in the first and early second trimesters of pregnancy demonstrated that the fetus exhibits all the components of the adult ECG waveform at an early stage of gestation (Easby, 1934; Heard, Burkley and Schaefer, 1936).

By 1941, Mann and Bernstein described in detail the optimal placement of external electrodes to the abdomen to obtain the FECG signal. Their statement that the amplifier electrocardiograph has now succeeded in eliminating much of the outside electrical and mechanical interferences which have been so disturbing to early workers exhibited perhaps unwarranted optimism, but in a report of 40 recordings, they were able to detect the fetal signal on 36 occasions. Furthermore, they demonstrated that the abdominal leads provided the best technique for obtaining the signal and that FECGs could be demonstrated as early as the 169th day of pregnancy. This was the earliest gestational age at which a signal had been recorded. The authors also noted that it was possible to observe temporary changes in rate corresponding to sinus arrhythmia, perhaps the first published observation on baseline variability. It is interesting to note that one of their conclusions stated that "... so far, sex cannot be prognosticated. Conclusions from a larger study will soon be forthcoming!"

In the same year, Dressler and Moskowitz developed a method of simultaneous phonocardiography and fetal electrocardiography. In a study on 40 women, they concluded with perhaps an element of hyperbole that "it is obvious from our results, that the study of the fetal heart by the fetal electrocardiogram and stethogram, either separately or simultaneously, is the only method available at present for an accurate assessment of fetal life." They observed that a negative waveform indicated a vertex presentation and a positive waveform, a breech presentation. They also noted that the reasons for failing to obtain a signal were a nervous mother, a small fetus, maternal tachycardia and possibly fetal sinus arrythmia.

The continuing use of a high-pass filter meant that the descriptions of work on the fetal ECG at this time was almost entirely dedicated to the recognition of the QRS waveform and most authors ignored the issue of filtering until this was acknowledged by Smyth in 1953. He stated that high-pass filtering up to a level of 30 Hz (−3 dB cut-off) had been widely used in systems used to record the fetal ECG and that at this level, the P and T waves would be completely obliterated. All of these studies were based on abdominal electrodes until the work of Smyth in 1953, and all work in this field was therefore hampered by the problems of using an inefficient system of signal acquisition and technical problems with both amplification and filtering.

Early Observations of the P&T Waves

By 1953, Smyth reported the next major step by developing an electrode that could be attached directly to the presenting part of the fetus. He used an intrauterine silver wire applied to the fetus and demonstrated that the fetal heart potential against unwanted potentials was improved by a factor of five as compared with the signal obtained from the abdominal electrodes (see Fig. 1.2). Examination of this paper shows little evidence of the P&T wave configuration.

In 1954, Davis and Meares described the use of a Grass electro-encephalograph and a multilead system that included abdominal and vaginal leads. No reference is made to the filtering characteristics of the electro-encephalograph but samples from recordings obtained from a 19-week fetus purportedly show the presence of a complete fetal electrocardiogram with a P wave, QRS complex and T wave. The recordings are by no means convincing. The studies by Southern (1957) used abdominal electrodes but concentrated on the P wave and the PR interval where it was possible to obtain measurements. An example of the recording obtained is shown in Fig. 1.3.

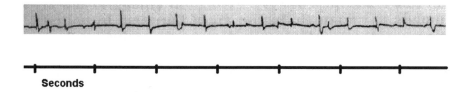

Seconds

Fig. 1.2. The first recording of the fetal ECG obtained with a silver-wire electrode in the amniotic sac (reprinted with permission from Smyth, 1953; copyright © The Lancet Ltd.).

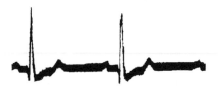

Fig. 1.3. Prenatal FECG obtained using maternal abdominal leads (reprinted with permission from Southern, 1957; copyright © Mosby, Inc.).

The study again was disadvantaged by the use of filters that provided low frequency cut-offs and may therefore have distorted P&T wave characteristics. Nevertheless, the data produced by measuring the PR interval and the QRS duration are probably valid within the constraints of the methodology and these measurements were related to oxygen saturation in the umbilical venous and arterial blood. Southern reported that diminished oxygen saturation was associated with bradycardia, prolonged PR interval which was probably a direct consequence of the fetal heart rate and a widened QRS complex. Changes with the T wave and ST segment were said to be characterised by depression of the ST segment and isoelectric or inverted T waves.

In 1956, Sureau produced data using a direct intrauterine electrode in labour but was unable to demonstrate any effects of labour on the FECG. Kaplan and Toyama (1958) used a cardiac catheterisation electrode placed inside the amniotic sac in apposition to the fetus following rupture of the membranes. In 12 cases, they were able to define characteristics of the time intervals. These values for the PQ interval differ slightly from those of Southern. Sureau (1956) also published intrapartum recordings of the FECG using a direct application electrode and these three studies represent the major technical advances that occurred in the 1950s and which laid the groundwork for the future of fetal electrocardiography.

The rather mixed and conflicting results in these reports highlight the continuing technical problems at that time but they also began to illustrate the difficulties related to signal processing and interpretation that were not really to see resolution for another 20 years. It was, however, at this stage that the use of this technology began to split into two different pathways. Because early studies on the FECG did not show any obvious and easily discernable changes in the waveform, emphasis switched to heart rate which was already embedded in the clinical literature as a standard part of management in the delivery suite. Intermittent auscultation with prescribed sampling intervals features in the standard protocols for intrapartum care and, therefore, there was a ready acceptance of electronic techniques that would simplify and make available continuous recordings of fetal heart rate. There is a mass of literature about the evolution, acceptance and partial rejection of cardiotocography and it is not the fundamental purpose of this book to address these issues. Some reference will be made to the subject at the end of this chapter. The second pathway was the improvement of the technology that has allowed continuous evaluation of the fetal ECG waveform and it is that topic which forms the basis of this work.

The P Wave and the QRS Complex

In a series of seminal papers written in the early 1960s, Hon and his coworkers set about attempting to resolve some of the fundamental difficulties that beset previous studies in this field. Having introduced a scalp clip that enabled direct application of an electrode to the fetus during labour, he set about solving the problems of noise reduction. This was to be partly resolved by using an 8–50 Hz filter which had the disadvantage of potentially obliterating the P&T waves. To enhance the signal-to-noise ratio, Hon and Lee (1963) recorded the FECG on magnetic tape and then played the tape back at 15 inches per second. Having amplified the signal to a 6 volts peak-to-peak level, they fed the tape into a pulse generator that put in a signal marker at a fixed time before the QRS complex and used the signal to trigger the computer to average the signal. Signal-to-noise ratios steadily improved as the number of computations was increased. It was apparent that the clarity of the signal enabled a clear exhibition of the P wave but the definition of the T wave was poor. Furthermore, optimal signal was achieved with an average of 50 computations, and whilst this only represents 20 seconds in real time, it may have been sufficient to mask short-term changes. In retrospect, it was probably the filtering that turned out to be the major disadvantage. Nevertheless, the use of a CAT computer in the analysis of the FECG did greatly improve the signal-to-noise ratio and it did uncover the FECG baseline and reveal P&T waves and the S–T segment changes as shown in Fig. 1.4.

This was a remarkable technical achievement and was at least ten years ahead of its time. These authors went on to enhance the technology by improving display and storage techniques (Hon and Lee, 1965) but the fundamental problem of filtering meant that much clinical information was lost. Furthermore, the clinician was left with the problems of eyeballing the waveform. Despite this work and earlier studies on the fetuses of pregnant dogs (Kaneoka *et al.*, 1961, Romney *et al.*, 1963), the fetal ECG appeared

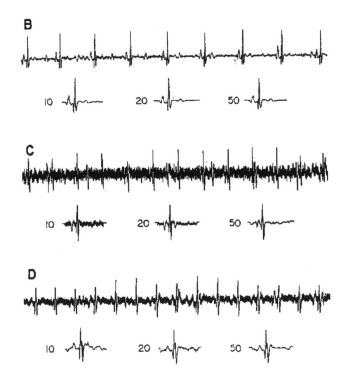

Fig. 1.4. Reduction of noise by computer averaging of the FECG (reprinted from Hon and Lee, 1963; copyright © Mosby, Inc.).

to be singularly resistant to change although there is evidence in the data of Hon and Lee (1963) that fetal hypoxia was associated with peaked, (biphasic) or inverted P waves and shortened PR intervals. This was a remarkable study on 22 cases of perinatal death where 9 infants eventually produced tracings that were suitable for evaluation. Four of these infants were anencephalic and it is therefore difficult to be certain to what degree the regulation of the fetal heart in these cases relates to the FECG obtained from a complete fetus. Four infants were premature and only one was at term. In this study, the authors pointed out some of the artefacts that occur in non-averaged data. Prominent fetal P waves were noted at recordings obtained using abdominal leads but these changes were shown to be associated with coincidence of the maternal T wave. Enlarged P waves were noted as well as being peaked in two anencephalic fetuses, and in the one normal full-term fetus, P waves were seen to be biphasic and the PR intervals were shortened. This study was far advanced for its time but the 8–50 Hz filtering may still have modified the P&T waveforms and, as demonstrated at a later stage, PR interval has to be interpreted in relation to the R–R interval or heart rate if it is to be of any significance. Changes in the ST segment and the morphology of the T wave, by analogy with the changes seen in adult ischaemic heart disease, would seem to have been the most attractive option in studies on fetal asphyxia but in reality they have turned out to be much more difficult to interpret in the fetus using a single lead system. Using a filter system of 8–50 Hz, the ST segment and T wave would merge and make satisfactory interpretation very difficult. In their paper on the dying fetus, Hon and Lee showed depression of the ST segment and inverted T waves, and in one case, they demonstrated what appeared to be biphasic T waves but these changes were observed in the agonal stages of life in an anencephalic fetus, as shown in Fig. 1.5.

Larks and Larks (1966) appeared to recognise the difficulties with filtering in that they used a bandwidth of 0.1–100 Hz. However, most of their work was dedicated to studies on the QRS complex and on vector-cardiography, and because their work is entirely based on the use of abdominal electrodes, there is little reference to the P&T waves. In a study on 84 subjects in labour, Larks and Longo (1962) did suggest that morphological changes of the ST segment "should be interpreted as a signal suggesting an

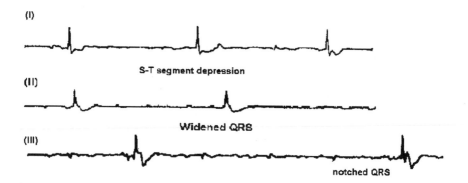

Fig. 1.5. Terminal stages of a FECG recorded from a 39-week anencephalic fetus showing widening of the QRS complex and dissociation of the P wave (reprinted with permission from Hon and Lee, 1963; copyright © Mosby, Inc.).

unfavourable fetal environment." They did not actually describe the nature of the changes, and in looking at the figures in this paper, it is difficult to see how they arrived at that particular conclusion. In a further publication in the same year, Larks and Anderson studied a further nine cases in labour and concluded that the ST segment depression or elevation was frequently associated with apparent "intrauterine and neonatal difficulties." It is difficult to evaluate these data because there is no consistent description of fetal condition at birth, and because even allowing for the improvement of quality in their recordings, the tracings are all obtained from the use of abdominal electrodes. Kendall *et al.* (1964) used a technique of fetal radio-electrocardiography concentrated on the ST segment changes, but because of filtering used in their studies, the T waves were not visible and it is therefore difficult to place any weight on this particular observation. In an extensive review of fetal electrocardiography up to 1966, Shenker concluded that whilst the FECG was valuable in investigating heart rate, the main clinical value lies in the diagnosis of fetal life and of multiple pregnancies. What he failed to appreciate at this time was that, with the exception of the works by Larks, most of the filter systems used had largely obliterated the P&T waveforms. Further attempts were made to characterise the FECG changes in controlled human and animal experiments by Gennser *et al.* (1968) and subsequently Gelli and Gyulai (1969). These studies showed lengthening of the PR or PQ intervals and ST segment and T wave inversion although this was only seen in 50% of animals despite severe asphyxia. The final paper in the saga of inappropriate filtering came out in 1971 when Davidsen, using high-pass filters and comparing the ECG and FHR changes in labour, concluded that the FECG was a poor indicator of fetal welfare during labour.

Observations on the FECG Waveform in the 1970s with Appropriate Filtering

In a study of intrapartum fetal ECGs obtained from scalp electrodes and measured against scalp blood and cord blood acid–base measurements, Symonds (1971) showed that lengthening occurred in the QT interval corrected for heart rate and that there was evidence that the QT interval was prolonged and the T wave inverted in the presence of increasing acidosis. It was also suggested that these changes were associated with high plasma potassium levels and possibly intracellular potassium loss as a result of the difference in plasma K^+ levels between maternal and fetal plasma in the presence of fetal acidosis due to asphyxia. The measurements in the study were all made by hand on the raw data and were therefore subject to measurement error although each measurement was obtained from a stable segment of recording and was the average of measurements taken from six sequential waveforms.

Further animal experiments on the exteriorised fetal lamb by Pardi *et al.* (1971) showed that a controlled reduction of oxygen tension to 0.8–1.9 kPa was associated with prolongation of the PQ interval and elevation of the ST segment and T wave height in the mature fetus. Rather similar findings were demonstrated by Myers in pregnant monkeys in 1972 using maternal aortic compression showing fetal ST segment and T wave elevation. None of these studies recognised the relationship between heart rate and the PQ and RR interval. The study by Yeh *et al.* in 1974 on fetal baboons was based on cord compression experiments and was largely directed at heart rate changes. However, the results in this work showed that complete atrioventricular block was seen in 6 of the 16 animals examined and that the PR interval became prolonged during the episodes of bradycardia. Cord compression is a very specific model in this type of study which also produces major cardiovascular effects and is therefore only analogous to those forms of asphyxia in the fetus that are directly related to cord compression. In the human subject, Roemer *et al.* (1972) studied the acid–base changes in relation to the FECG but it seems high-pass filtering was used in this study and, therefore, the results are difficult to interpret. Lee and Blackwell (1974) used a 3–200 Hz bandwidth and showed that the PR interval and the corrected QT were shortened with variable decelerations and the PR interval was shortened in the presence of fetal tachycardia. The relationship between PR and R–R has proven to be of critical significance in later studies but it looked like at this stage that animal data was not consistent in fetal asphyxia as far as the PR interval was concerned. However, in terms of the shape of the waveform, the ST segment was raised as was the T wave height, whereas in human studies, the data on the FECG waveform tended to favour a prolonged QT interval and depression or inversion of the T wave and ST segment.

Pardi *et al.* (1974) returned to averaging techniques in a study of 234 labours in which the taped FECG was converted into digital form and the digitized complexes were summed, averaged and converted back into the analogue form. Findings were compared against scalp blood measurements but the major interest in this study was to compare changes against the heart rate pattern as the index of fetal distress. It is interesting that biphasic or absent P waves and shortened PQ intervals were noted in the presence of variable decelerations, a finding that was to be repeated in 1995 by Mohajer *et al.* This appeared to be an artefact of using averaging techniques as the true explanation appears to be the dissociation of the P wave from the QRS complex as a result of atrioventricular heart block. Westgate *et al.* in 1998 also demonstrated that, when subjected to cord occlusion, the fetal ECG showed evidence of second degree heart block and this was more common when the heart rate fell below 70 beats/minute, an experimental observation that directly confirmed the observations in the human fetus. In 17 out of 35 late decelerations, Pardi *et al.* (1974) showed that there was ST segment depression or shift and that there was generally an increase in T wave amplitude. Occasionally, in the late decelerations, there was T wave inversion. Hioki (1975), in a similar study, used averaged waveforms in a sampling mode and showed depressed ST segments and shortened PR and QT intervals, but the comparisons were made against decelerations, and in view of the known modest relationship of these indices with acid–base status, it is difficult to interpret the significance of this study.

By 1980, the only study that had systematically examined specific alterations in the fetal ECG with both intrapartum and cord blood acid–base and electrolyte measurements was published by Symonds in 1971.

New Methods of Signal Processing in the 1980s

The rapid improvements that occurred in signal processing and computer technology that began in the 1960s accelerated in the 1980s. Two groups in Göteborg and Nottingham worked on signal isolation and measurement techniques that enabled real time and accurate quantification of the changes in the fetal ECG. The group in Göteborg concentrated on waveform configuration and in particular the ST segment and T wave height. The Nottingham group worked on a complete data acquisition system but concentrated on the P wave and PR interval as well as the T wave configuration. Their studies were all initially on the human fetus. In Sweden, Rosen and Gjellmer (1975) induced asphyxia in fetal lambs by maternal aortic compression and showed an absolute increase in T wave amplitude with increasing hypoxia, and subsequently, the same group (Rosen and Isaksson, 1976) demonstrated depletion of glycogen and creatinine phosphate in the myocardium of the fetus. In 1976, Rosen *et al.* showed an increase in T wave amplitude in relation to metabolic acidosis and in the presence of increased lactacidosis. The T wave changes preceded the fall in fetal arterial pressure and thus predated the onset of myocardial failure.

These observations were essentially repeated by Greene *et al.* (1982) in chronically instrumented lambs *in utero* and the increase in T wave amplitude in relation to myocardial hypoxia was confirmed but they could not demonstrate these findings following adrenaline infusion. These observations were pursued in a group of 46 patients who were observed by CTG and by intermittent measurement of the T/QRS ratio (Lilja *et al.*, 1985). A linear correlation was demonstrated between cord venous blood lactate levels and the T/QRS ($r = 0.58$, $p < 0.01$) and there was evidence that abnormal CTGs were much commoner than abnormal changes in the T/QRS ratio. In the data presentation in this paper, there is one outlying number in the data that reports a T/QRS value close to 1.0 and it is possible that this has a significant impact on the slope of the line and on the *r* value. The authors also reported marked T wave and ST segment changes as seen through periods of bradycardia and variable decelerations. Hökegärd *et al.* in Göteborg, reporting observations in the neonate in 1978, also demonstrated high T/QRS ratios where delivery had been preceded by abnormal CTGs and where the infants were depressed at birth with low Apgar scores. In 1986, Jenkins *et al.* in Nottingham, using a technique that was developed in Nottingham, described a comparative study of the fetal ECG in a group of 14 fetuses where the clinical and biochemical measurements were normal, and in 10 infants where the mean cord arterial pH was 7.11. The method used involved recognition of the signal by a DEC LSI-11/23 computer and enhancement of the signal-to-noise ratio of the waveform by a software-generated time-coherent filtering process. Non-repetitive transient features were filtered out and line fitting to the complex allowed accurate measurement of the ST signal and T wave height. The technique allows real time analysis. The conclusion from this study was that there was a highly significant difference between the two groups with elevation of both the ST segment and the T wave height in the acidotic group. Newbold *et al.* (1989), again using data averaging techniques, studied a group of 25 women with normal pregnancies. The data were obtained during labour. Using an isoelectric line set between the pre-P wave region, they demonstrated variations from 4–23% in the T/QRS ratios in these normal infants with a mean of 10%. They also showed that the effect of contractions on the T/QRS ratio was inconsistent. It must be said, however, that these were normal subjects and that the maximum values fell below the range for abnormal infants reported by Rosen and others. Murray (1986) in Nottingham investigated an observation from a PhD thesis (1982) in Nottingham by J.M. Family. Family applied a cross-correlation technique to a large number of variables measured from the FECG and identified that in normal labour, there was a negative relationship between PR interval and heart rate. Murray (1986) pursued this observation in an extensive study and showed that the negative correlation changed to a positive correlation when the fetus became acidotic. He also showed that P wave duration had a negative correlation with noradrenaline levels in the cord venous blood at the time of delivery and that there was a strong negative correlation between the cord venous blood levels and the PR interval. He reported his data in this paper on the RR interval rather than heart rate, and under these circumstances, there is a positive relationship between the PR interval and the R–R′ interval with *r* values up to 0.95. In the fetuses developing acidosis with a low pH, the relationship between PR and RR became negative. However, using this parameter by itself, it was clear that there was considerable overlap between the normal pH range and the low pH group. Discrimination was further enhanced if a shift in the ST segment by more than 5% in relation to the QRS complex was noted as this enhanced the effect of using the ECG parameters in recognising fetal acidosis. It must also be pointed out, as originally observed by Symonds in 1971, that like the adult heart, there is a strong correlation between RR interval and QT interval. Murray's work included studies from 155 women in labour that would generally be considered as a high-risk population. The mean duration of labour was seven hours so that his studies on the PR/FHR relationship using the Nottingham FECG monitor were the most extensive published at that time.

Clinical Trials and Observations in Recent Studies

Newbold *et al.* (1991) reported a study on 105 women in labour and classified the patients according to the pattern of the FHR. They also measured acid–base and lactate values in cord arterial samples at the time of delivery. They examined the T/QRS ratio in early and late labour and showed overall that there was a small decrease in the T/QRS ratio from 11–5% in 11 fetuses with an abnormal FHR pattern. Eight infants were born with a moderate degree of acidosis and four were born in poor condition with no evidence of acidosis. None of those infants had a T/QRS ratio outside the normal range and, on this basis, the authors concluded that T/QRS changes were sometimes transient and that "although the proponents of T/QRS ratio measurement have emphasised the shortcomings of FHR monitoring, it seems unlikely that the T/QRS ratio alone will be an adequate substitute."

Several further studies appeared in 1992. Murphy *et al.* (1992) published a further descriptive study of the use of the FECG waveform in labour on 86 high-risk pregnancies. Using the Göteborg system known as the ST segment analyser (STAN), they measured T/QRS ratios and the intrapartum CTG in relation to umbilical artery pH at birth and Apgar scores. Their data indicated that there was no correlation between T/QRS and the Apgar score at one minute and five minutes but this is not surprising in view of the generally "soft" nature of the Apgar score in expressing fetal damage from asphyxia. However, it was observed that, in the 16 infants with Apgar score < 7 at one minute, only three had a mean T/QRS above the stated normal range, i.e. about 0.25. There was a weak correlation between T/QRS and cord artery base deficit but none with pH. The mean one hour T/QRS ratio at any of the three stages listed (4, 8 and 10 cms cervical dilatation) was above 0.25 in only one of the 11 infants with acidosis, although in only four infants was the acidosis metabolic in origin. There was no significant correlation between the mean one hour T/QRS at 8 and 10 cms and umbilical artery pH or base deficit.

A further study was reported by MacLachlan *et al.* (1992) on 113 women in labour at term. Again, the main outcome measures were the correlation of the fetal T/QRS with pH values from scalp blood sampling and at birth in the umbilical artery blood. The predictive values of the CTG and T/QRS were compared. T/QRS ratios did not correlate with fetal scalp blood pH. However, at delivery, the correlation between T/QRS and umbilical artery pH was significant ($n = 93$, $r = 0.349$, $p < 0.001$). Despite this result, the authors concluded that a raised T/QRS ratio had a considerably lower detection rate for fetal acidaemia during labour than a pathological CTG. Clearly, the consensus beginning to emerge from these studies was that the T/QRS was not providing any significant benefit in predicting fetal acidosis whilst being firmly based on a good scientific foundation in both animal and human studies. The question that remained to be answered was whether this technology could have a significant impact on management by reducing the level of unnecessary intervention that has characterised the use of CTG, but to reduce intervention as well as improving the prediction of acidosis. In July 1992, Westgate *et al.* reported a large randomised trial of cardiotocography alone or with ST waveform analysis. They assigned 1200 women to the groups well before the onset of labour and assessed neonatal outcome by umbilical cord blood gas analysis, Apgar score, resuscitation needed and postnatal course. A total of 606 patients were included in the CTG group and 615 in the ST + CTG group.

There was no significant difference between the two groups in terms of the frequency of FBS sampling. However, there was a significant reduction in intervention rates in the form of delivery by Caesarean section or forceps delivery (CTG 19% versus ST + CTG 5%). There was one baby in each group that exhibited birth asphyxia. Of the babies with cord pH values below 7.15, 58 occurred in the CTG group and 59 in the ST + CTG group. These babies were described as showing mild or moderate acidosis although one of these infants had a cord artery pH of 6.87 and one had a cord artery pH of 7.03 and required ventilation for 48 hours. Both these infants were in the CTG group. Ten babies in the CTG group had pH values < 7.05 and seven babies in the ST + CTG group showed similar values. This was the first large randomised trial to use ECG parameters for clinical management and provided evidence of benefit in terms of reduced operative intervention. This was effectively the last large study performed so far on the STAN technique although further studies are now underway.

Following the earlier work of Murray (1986), almost a decade elapsed before the next major publications appeared on work on the PR interval during labour. Then in 1995, Mohajer *et al.* in a joint study between the University of Nottingham and the Chinese University of Hong Kong published a further clinical and retrospective study on 132 subjects selected on the basis that they were high-risk pregnancies. The relationship between the PR interval and FHR is described as the Conduction Index and it was known that, whilst there was a proven relationship between PR & FHR which changed from negative to positive in the acidotic infant, the relationship was subject to short-term fluctuations which could often be stimulated by touching the fetal head or by procedures such as scalp blood sampling. These short-term changes were probably based on catecholamine surges. However, to make allowance for the temporal basis of these changes, it was necessary to develop an index that would provide a cumulative expression of the conduction index over the course of the labour. In this study, the data for the PR interval and the FHR were subject to Z-transformation and were then used to calculate the total number of waveforms in excess of two standard deviations above the mean estimated for the whole labour. This is addressed in more detail in Chapter 7. This was described as the ratio index and clearly was initially only applicable in this study on the basis of retrospective analysis. Nevertheless, the study showed that, in an analysis of 132 labours, the ratio index ranged from 0–10% of the labour time and there was a significant negative correlation with cord artery pH ($p < 0.001$) and a positive relationship with cord lactate, hypoxanthine and log noradrenaline (all at $p < 0.001$). This demonstrated a potential new quantitative approach to fetal management in labour. The procedure was modified to a "running mean" for calculation of the ratio index and, based on observational data, a ratio index $> 4\%$ was found to correlate with metabolic acidosis in the fetus. Reed *et al.* (1996) reported on a further study of 265 women who were managed according to conventional CTG monitoring. The condition of the fetus at delivery was assessed from cord blood acid–base status in both cord venous and cord arterial blood. Further assessment involved Apgar scores at 1, 5 and 10 minutes and the need for admission to the Neonatal Intensive Care Unit. All labours were recorded and a comparison was then made retrospectively between management on the CTG as actually happened compared with management as would have happened using a conduction index persistently positive for ≥ 20 minutes and a ratio index of $> 4\%$.

Thirty-six infants (14.6%) had a cord arterial pH ≤ 7.15 and 52 fetuses (21.1%) had an Apgar score ≤ 7 at one minute. For the hypothetical exercise, intervention was only indicated if two of the three parameters (FHR, CI and RI) were positive. There were no admissions to NNICU for birth asphyxia. This is a complex study and suffered from the disadvantages that one arm of the study was retrospective. Nevertheless, it showed that the addition of PR interval assessment would have reduced the number of fetal scalp blood samples from 85.5–26.8% and that the proportion of "missed acidosis" would have fallen from 8.5–4.5%.

Van Wijngaarden *et al.* (1996) studied changes in the PR interval and heart rate in fetal lambs subjected to controlled fetal hypoxaemia and demonstrated that the same changes occurred in the conduction index in the fetal lamb as had been observed in the human fetus, and that the conduction index reverted to a negative correlation when the hypoxaemia was reversed. Of the 16 animals used in the final analysis, 12 showed a statistically significant change from a predominantly negative pattern during normoxaemia to a predominantly positive pattern during hypoxaemia. Two cases showed a trend towards the same pattern and two showed no change.

The first randomised study in management on the basis of these observations was reported by Van Wijngaarden *et al.* (1996). A randomised study of CTG versus CTG + CI was performed on 214 women. The study showed that there was a significant reduction in fetal blood sampling in the FECG group (3.53; $p < 0.01$) and that the samples taken in the FECG group were more likely to be normal, or conversely, that there were fewer cases of missed acidosis in the FECG group (9% versus 4.8%). This study shows considerable promise for this technique and needs to be subjected to further large randomised studies. It is addressed again in Chapter 7.

The QRS Complex

Far less effort has been concentrated on the fetal QRS complex apart from the uses of the R wave to measure the RR interval and heart rate. Although most of the early studies are confused by the problems of filtering, it is clear from the literature that the QRS complex was the easiest signal to recognise and that there are a limited number of features that can actually be measured. Easby in 1934 measured the QRS duration from a 4 1/2-month fetus that had been removed from the uterus after hysterectomy and reported a QRS duration of 0.04 second, and Vara and Niemineva (1951) obtained direct readings at hysterectomy with the fetus *in situ* and demonstrated values of 0.02–0.03 second for QRS duration.

Although Smyth (1953) was the first investigator to apply a lead directly to the fetus *in utero* and to demonstrate the enhanced quality of the ECG recording, he did not report any measurements on the QRS complex, and the first direct physiological measurements were made by Sureau in 1956 when he reported a QRS duration of 0.05 second and later in 1960, between 0.034 and 0.052 second. Southern produced an extensive report in 1957 using abdominal electrodes and using low-frequency cut-offs which may have impaired the recognition of P&T waves. He nevertheless produced data on the QRS duration that were in the range of 0.02–0.04 second. He then examined the values obtained in 22 women where there was clinical evidence of fetal distress as judged by the presence of fetal bradycardia and the passage of thick meconium. In this study, he reported that the average duration of the QRS complex was prolonged. He also studied 20 patients with hypertension in pregnancy but was unable to show any differences in the QRS duration. However, he did suggest that post-mature fetuses exhibited a QRS duration of 0.05 second. There is no statistical analysis of the data and it is difficult to draw any conclusions from the results. Nevertheless, this was the first systematic study where an author set out to quantify FECG measurements in relation to specific maternal and fetal complications.

Southern postulated from his study that alterations in the P wave, PR interval, QRS voltage, ST segment and T waves are present in the prenatal fetal electrocardiogram in association with reduced oxygenation of the fetus. Further studies using a scalp lead were reported by Kaplan and Toyama in

1963. They showed QRS durations between 0.034 and 0.052 second but did not come to any conclusion about the value of these measurements in a clinical context. The difficulty about these studies generally was technical and future developments were therefore directed towards the use of the QRS complex as a trigger in counting the heart rate and for the shape of the QRS waveform to indicate the polarity of the fetus. It was apparent that further advances would not occur until the signal-to-noise ratio could be improved and where very small time measurements could be machine-read rather than by manual measurement. In a report published in 1962, Lamkee *et al.* stated, somewhat unfairly, that up to this time, only the work of Hon and Hess "can be credited with making really significant contributions to the field" — a judgement that seemed rather harsh in view of many excellent contributions up to that time. These authors then produced a report of a method that they claimed was "based on a special vector approach to electrocardiography". This method described the placement of abdominal electrodes but the claims were based on a false premise because of failing to understand the manner by which the fetal signal reaches the abdominal wall. The low-frequency cut-off was stated to be between 0.15 to 1.5 cycles per second. This was an antenatal study and the mean duration for the QRS duration was shown to vary from 0.02 second in early frequency to 0.04 second near term. These data were validated many years later using signal averaging techniques.

Hon and Lee, in two publications in 1963 and 1964, described the averaging methods developed to enhance signal-to-noise ratio, but despite these improvements, the actual time intervals still had to be measured by hand. Despite a further report by Lee and Hon in 1963 on a series of seven cases in which there was notching or splitting and widening of the R wave, the authors concluded that spontaneous variations in the R wave amplitude were not rare during labour and that these morphological changes did not indicate an adverse fetal environment. In their paper on the dying fetus (1963), the same authors concluded that, whilst there was on occasions evidence of a wandering pacemaker and widened QRS complexes, these changes were not consistent and were generally agonal.

These observations were reinforced in the studies by Larks and Longo (1962) of 84 subjects in labour. They concluded that widening of QRS complexes and ST segment changes and bizarre changes in morphology were generally late and were consistent with terminal fetal ECG activity. These findings were again reinforced in further publications by the same authors on the abnormal fetal electrocardiograph in 1962, and they suggested that a new series of grades could be identified ranging through changes of "slight significance", "alert" and "concern". The last category described the emergence of pronounced or persistent bradycardia in early to middle labour but makes no mention of the morphology or duration of the fetal QRS. Subsequently, in 1963, Larks reported further examples of morphological changes occurring during labour in ten patients and suggested that not all attention should be directed to heart rate alone as there were instances of fetal QRS waveform changes and major arrhythmias.

Nevertheless, because of the difficulty of assessing morphological changes generally, it was not until the 1980s that interest reemerged on the duration of the QRS complex. In 1986, Pardi and his colleagues published a paper entitled "The intraventricular conduction time of fetal heart in pregnancies with suspected fetal growth retardation". This study was based on the premise that fetal growth retardation was associated with a reduction in the weight of the fetal heart in fetal lambs where growth had been impaired by the gradual embolisation of the utero-placental vascular bed. The study in 1986 was performed on 68 pregnant women who were suspected by ultrasound evaluation to be carrying growth-retarded fetuses. The method involved the use of abdominal leads on the mother to obtain the fetal ECG, but by this time, the technology had become considerably more sophisticated.

The method used in this study and reported in 1980 by Brambati and Pardi was initially used to establish conduction times in normal pregnancies, and subsequently in 1981, in pregnancies complicated by Rh haemolytic disease. The fetal signal is detected from electrodes placed on the maternal abdomen. The maternal R wave is erased and the digitized fetal complexes are summed, averaged and converted back into analogue form. An average of 50 complexes produced readable ECG traces, and the QRS duration was measured. This study showed that there was a highly significant relationship between the QRS duration and birth weight ($r = 0.69$, $p < 0.001$). In 56 of the 68 fetuses, the fetal ECG was recorded within one week before delivery. All but one of the normally grown fetuses had QRS values that lay within the previously established normal range. Forty-seven infants were shown to be small for dates, and the relationship between QRS duration and severity of growth retardation was statistically significant. Of the 11 fetuses that had a QRS duration value below 4SD, nine had birth weights that were below the tenth percentile.

In their study on a large series of uncomplicated pregnancies, Brambati and Pardi (1980) reported abdominal fetal ECG recordings from 421 women and established that the relationship between gestational age and the QRS duration followed a curve corresponding to a second-degree polynomial on data collected throughout pregnancy. The relationship between birth weight in 78 fetuses and QRS duration where measurements were made within one week of delivery was linear and highly significant ($r = 0.82$, $p < 0.001$). These authors failed to establish any significant sex difference although the duration tended to be greater in male fetuses. Their mean values varied from 28.7–53.0 milliseconds. A further study published in 1991 by Morgan and Symonds on intrapartum ECGs showed a significant difference in QRS duration between male and female infants with a longer time interval in the male infants. The study also showed that the QRS duration was unaffected by contractions. There was a positive correlation with birth weight as demonstrated in the studies of Brambati and Pardi.

The QRS duration is small and, until computer analysis of the waveform became available, it was difficult to measure with the degree of accuracy that was necessary to demonstrate any differences induced by events or by inherent factors. Furthermore, within the physiological range of fetal activity, intraventricular conduction time of the fetal heart tends to be surprisingly constant and the voltage of the signal is variable depending on the nature of the electrodes used. The signal duration also appears to be unaffected by heart rate, uterine contractions and the presence of the cord around the neck.

Vectorcardiography

In 1965, Larks reported studies on the fetal ECG that were based on the concept that it was possible to determine the electrical axis of the fetal heart in signals obtained from the abdominal wall of the mother. These fetal signals appear to be similar to lead II QRS in the neonate and clearly are influenced by the presentation of the fetus. The mechanism by which the waveform spreads from the fetal heart to the abdominal wall remains in dispute. Workers, such as Kahn in 1963 and Roche and Hon in 1965, suggested that the alteration of the position of the electrodes on the maternal abdomen made little difference to the shape of the waveform and that the conduction of the impulse was either through the oronasal cavity of the fetus or through the umbilical cord.

Larks and Larks worked on the basis that it was possible to measure the electrical axis of the fetal heart and that the projection upon lead II was mathematically related to the electrical axis vector × the sine of the angle which the electrical axis forms with the 150 degree line.

They calculated that the value of the fetal complex was the net algebraic sum of R&S normalised to a scale of 10. On this basis, they calculated the electrical axis of the heart and demonstrated that the normal range lay from 100–160 degrees and that values less than 100 degrees were defined as left-axis shift whilst values greater than 160 degrees were defined as right-axis shift. In their discussion of this work, they suggested that there is increased right-axis deviation in those infants subjected to hypoxia and believed this situation to be similar to that of children born in the Andes at high altitude where the QRS axis remains between 135–140 degrees after birth as compared with those born at sea level where the axis shifts to the left to around 90 degrees by three to six months. They also showed in a separate study (1966) that the mean value for the fetal cardiac axis at term is consistent with a relative right ventricular predominance and with relatively high right ventricular and pulmonary arterial pressures.

The problem with much of these data on axis measurement was that they were not measured against any quantifiable outcome criteria. In 1972, Symonds reported a study on 103 women in labour where the fetal ECG obtained by scalp electrode was compared with the neonatal ECG recorded within five hours after delivery. Changes in the R/S ratio in late labour were significantly related to changes in lead II of the neonatal electro-cardiogram. Using the method described by Larks to calculate electrical axis, the mean cardiac axis in early labour was +144.5°, and in late labour, it was +143°. The value in the neonate was +134°. The fetal values were then examined in relation to scalp blood pH and cord venous blood pH and plasma potassium values. Although the study is limited by the use of cord venous blood pH alone, there was a significant shift to the left in the presence of acidosis and hyperkalaemia and that the same axis shift was reflected in the neonatal ECG. It is perhaps surprising that although the calculation of cardiac axis on a single electrode has potential problems, no one has pursued this pathway which is, from a measurement point of view, simple and robust.

Fetal Cardiac Arrythmias

Cardiac arrythmias play an important part in the diagnosis of cardiac pathology in the adult but the processes involved in adult cardiac disease, with the exception of those based on congenital abnormalities, have little bearing on the effects induced by fetal hypoxia and fetal acidosis. Further, until recently, it has not been possible antenatally to obtain consistent recordings of P waves, and therefore, it has been difficult to interpret the nature of some arrythmias.

Heart block may present as profound fetal bradycardia, and may on occasions, lead to unnecessary intervention. However, the commonest arrhythmias tend to be supraventricular extrasystoles. In 1962, Hon and Huang documented a series of 25 arrythmias and missed beats of which 23 were of supraventricular origin and two were ventricular. The majority of these extrasystoles disappear immediately after birth but two persisted for 48 hours. There was no evidence that these arrythmias were associated with fetal compromise. Shenker published an extensive review of this subject in 1966 and concluded that fetal electrocardiography had little to contribute in the diagnosis of congenital heart disease. Various case reports continue to appear in the literature. Schneider *et al.* in 1977 reported a case of fetal trigeminal rhythm when these different heart rates were identified associated with premature beats occurring after every third beat. This child was normal at birth and subsequently returned to a normal sinus rhythm. Katz *et al.* in 1979 reported a case of congenital mitral and aortic stenosis that was diagnosed from the fetal electrocardiogram. Young *et al.* in the same year reported 15 cases of cardiac arrythmias noted during labour and estimated that the frequency of occurrence of arrythmias was 12.4/1000 monitored births. Most of these arrythmias were supraventricular in origin and commonly presented as atrial bigeminy and trigeminy. Two cases of ventricular arrhythmias were noted. All of these infants were normal at birth and it was concluded that these types of arrhythmia were of no clinical significance.

In a recent publication on computer analysis of the FECG, Mohajer and her colleagues (1995) examined the ECG in 15 fetuses during profound heart rate decelerations. In five cases, the appearances were those of sinus bradycardia and in one case, there was inversion of the P waves (Fig. 1.6). However, in seven cases, there was complete dissociation of the P waves from the QRS complex and the authors postulated that this represented a complete atrioventricular heart block, probably reflecting an effect of hypoxia on the bundle of His. The heart returned to a sinus rhythm as soon as the heart rate returned to normal.

Tachyarrhythmias

Very rapid impulses, apparently from the fetus, have been documented in the literature since the 1960s and have been a subject of some contention as regards to the origin of the signals. Bernstine (1961) took the view that very rapid complexes represented auricular fibrillation, flutter or paroxysmal tachycardias and these observations were reinforced in the publication by Muller-Schmid (1989). The issue was addressed by Reygaerts *et al.* (1961) who reported the occurrence of tachyarrhythmia in 22 cases and considered that all of these cases were artefacts. There are various possibilities that could explain very rapid impulses up to rates of 300–800 beats per minute but the most likely one appears to be that these impulses could be due to electromyograms. Whitfield (1966) reported a series of rapid impulses in 12 recordings from abdominal electrodes applied to seven patients including three recordings in labour. All the mothers eventually delivered normal infants. In some cases, the duration of the tachyarrhythmia was short-lived, but on three occasions, the impulses persisted throughout the entire recording lasting over one hour. The impulses varied at rates between 350–700 pulses/minute but were of low voltage. He pointed out that in three patients, he was able to initiate the signals by having the patients contract their muscles.

A

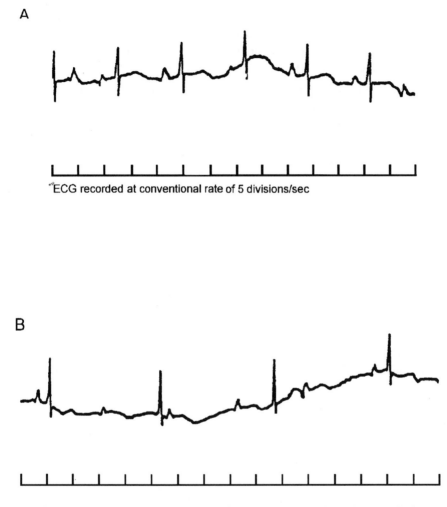

ECG recorded at conventional rate of 5 divisions/sec

B

Fig. 1.6. P wave area appears to diminish and disappear with profound bradycardia because of the dissociation of the P wave from the QRS complex (reprinted with permission from Mohajer *et al.*, 1995; copyright © BMJ Publishing Group).

He concluded that the impulses were maternal in origin "probably representing the summated potential of a small number of contracting motor units in the rectus abdominus muscle".

Despite these observations, there are genuine cases of fetal tachy-arrhythmias although these are usually at slower heart rates. Symonds (1972) reported a case where a persistent tachycardia around 190 beats per minute showed evidence of a nodal tachycardia with occasional impulses arising in the sino-auricular node. The changes were basically those seen in the presence of a wandering pacemaker.

The literature generally supports the belief that most cardiac arrhythmias are of no clinical significance. However, some abnormalities, particularly those associated with heart block, do have clinical implications.

The Use of Abdominal Electrodes

Until the 1960s, nearly all studies on fetal electrocardiogram were based on recordings obtained by the use of electrodes placed on the maternal abdomen. The information that was usable was almost entirely based on heart rate or the R–R′ interval or the QRS width. The one exception to this approach that appeared in the 1960s was the use of the QRS complex to perform vectorcardiography. The use of the abdominal fetal ECG for heart rate calculation was superceded by the emergence of Doppler ultrasound technology. FECG signals have a low voltage and are often obscured by electrical noise from other sources, so that the signal can be difficult to obtain and difficult to process if the maternal ECG is not removed.

However, the technology of signal recognition and isolation has moved forward substantially in the last decade and some reactivation of work on the abdominal FECG has begun to emerge. The work of Brambati and Pardi during the 1980s showed that it was possible, by cancelling the maternal ECG and averaging the fetal complex from recordings from the maternal abdomen, to isolate the complete complex. These authors used the signal to measure QRS width and, as previously mentioned, produced some very interesting observations on the relationship between weight in both normal and growth retarded infants in relationship to QRS duration. Curiously, this has never really been taken up as an observation and has not, with the exception of the paper from Morgan and Symonds, been repeated by other workers in this field. Furthermore, they used only the QRS complex and not the P wave on PR interval which was frequently demonstrated by their method.

Recently, Cicinelli and his coworkers (1994) reported the development of a multilead system of abdominal electrodes. His system simultaneously acquires signals from three space axes and allows real-time analysis of the signal. In recording signals in 140 women from 29–42 weeks of pregnancy, the QRS complex was detected in 93.6% of cases and a reliable evaluation of the P & QRS waves and of the ST interval could be achieved in 72.8% of recordings.

In 1996 Crowe and his colleagues also reported the development of an antenatal FECG analyser by using an isolated amplifier to obtain the signals, an analogue-to-digital converter card and a computer to process the digitised information. After elimination of the maternal ECG, a matched filter constructed from the FECG-QRS complex was used for coherent averaging of the entire complex and typically, signals were analysed over 15 seconds or some 30–40 impulses. The success rate was approximately 75% but the important aspect of this work was that it was able to present a complex suitable for line fitting and with clear features of the P and T waves as well as the QRS complex. Figure 1.7 shows a typical fetal waveform extracted by Crowe and his colleagues.

These studies now begin to point a way forward in obtaining and analysing signals from the maternal abdomen which have not previously been available and, once again, these studies indicate how intimately progress in this field is related to advances in computer and chip technology.

One additional method under investigation at the present time is the recognition of the fetal signal by changes in electromagnetic fields. Superconducting quantum interference device (SQUID) technology has been used by Quinn *et al.* (1994) and it was shown that it was possible to obtain a QRS complex in 67% of cases and that P&T waves, shown in Fig 1.8, could be demonstrated in over 70% of the cases where the QRS complex was seen.

At present, the equipment is expensive and cumbersome but it does potentially provide a technology that would avoid the windows of disappearing signals that characterise the use of abdominal electrodes, and it should reduce problems with background noise, although these difficulties can now largely be overcome using averaging techniques.

Maternal Thorax

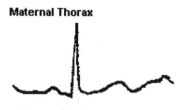

Magnified view of FECG

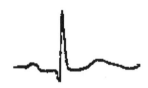

Averaged Maternal Thorax

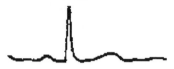

Enhanced FECG after group averaging

Abdominal Signal

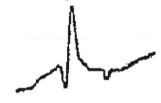

Enhanced FECG after group averaging

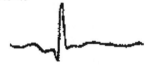

Enhanced FECG after group averaging

Averaged Abdominal Maternal Signal

Enhanced FECG after group averaging

FECG after subtraction of averaged maternal signal

Enhanced FECG after group averaging

Fig. 1.7. FECG signal obtained using averaged signals after removal of the maternal ECG. The quality of the signal depends on the number of signals averaged (reprinted with permission from Crowe *et al.*, 1996; copyright © Walter de Gruyter GmbH & Co. KG).

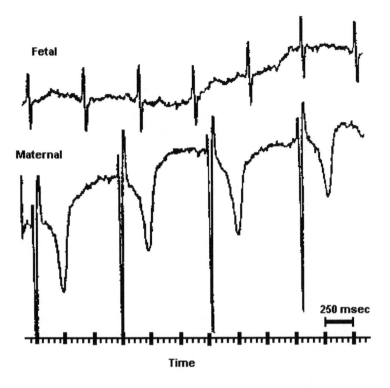

Fig. 1.8. Fetal magneto-cardiograph obtained at 40 weeks gestation without averaging using a neuromagnetometer placed 2 cm above the maternal abdomen (reprinted with permission from Quinn *et al.*, 1994; copyright © Blackwell Science Ltd.).

The R–R′ Interval and Fetal Heart Rate

It is not our intention to review the vast literature on R–R′ interval and fetal heart rate monitoring as this has been extensively covered in a range of publications, both review articles and books. Furthermore, much of the heart rate research has been based on Doppler ultrasound or phonocardiography and not on the use of the R wave in the fetal ECG. Nevertheless, the measurement of the R–R′ interval is important in the assessment of the heart rate and in establishing the baseline variability as well as beat-to-beat variability. It is our intention to discuss the use of the fetal QRS complex as it applies to heart rate and to the other time intervals in the FECG and to examine the difficulties with interpretation of heart rate which have been compounded by interobserver variability. The use of computer technology in the interpretation of fetal heart rate based on the use of the QRS complex offers some prospect of removing these inconsistencies.

It is interesting to note that most papers, where the interval between heart beats are used, are reported in terms of heart rate rather than R–R' interval. Consequently, all the original definitions by Hon (1968) described in his atlas are based on heart rate and not the R–R' interval. The current FIGO definition is also based on this information. Some of the most remarkable studies in this respect were published by Caldeyro-Barcia and his colleagues in 1966 where electrodes were inserted directly into the fetal buttocks. The impact of uterine contractions on the fetal heart rate derived from the fetal ECG were studied and descriptions of patterns of heart rate change similar to those described by Hon were produced.

The problem that causes high intervention rates is in part due to the variability in the scanning of analogue recordings by different observers.

Several groups of workers have now published extensively on the use of computers for pattern recognition. In particular, Maeda has developed a computer system for the assessment of the fetus by what he calls an actocardiogram and Dawes and other (1991) have developed computerised systems for the analysis of antenatal fetal heart rate. These systems allow for the establishment of accurate assessment of beat-to-beat and baseline variability as well as recognising accelerations and decelerations.

These studies and the possible way forward will be addressed in the relevant chapters in this book.

Chapter 2

FETAL ADAPTATION

What is Fetal Distress?

Fetal distress was first identified and associated with observations that preceded fetal death, and included the excessive increase or decrease of fetal movements, the passage of meconeum and the slowing of the fetal heart.

With increasing understanding of the metabolic and physiological consequences of hypoxia, the term fetal distress became linked to the presence of fetal acidosis and changes in fetal heart rate patterns (Haverkamp et al., 1979; Haesslein and Niswander, 1980). It was thought that fetal acidosis and the associated changes in fetal heart rate patterns reflected the severity of hypoxia (Myers et al., 1973), and hence the probability and severity of long-term adverse outcome for the fetus. The use of fetal and biochemical monitoring during labour was therefore thought to be capable of detecting fetal distress, and the intervention that follows would be capable of preventing long-term morbidity (Beard et al., 1971; Edington et al., 1975).

Experience showed that the earlier expectations from this technology could not be realised. Cases exhibiting signs of fetal distress were not always followed by subsequent morbidity (Steer, 1982; Parer and Livingston, 1990), and demonstrable signs of fetal distress during labour did not always precede the delivery of morbid newborns (Barela et al., 1983; Dennis et al., 1989; Gilstrap et al., 1989; Fee et al., 1990; Goldaber et al., 1991; Winkler et al., 1991; Goodwin et al., 1992).

This has led to an understanding that cellular damage in the fetus occurs not only during labour but also under a wide variety of circumstances at other times. Consequently, neither the presence nor absence of abnormal heart rate patterns during labour can exclude hypoxic damage already imposed or yet to occur.

Acute hypoxia provokes wide ranging physiological responses. These included adaptive changes in the pH and blood gases in the fetal blood, and the autonomic and cardiac responses to these changes. The presence of these signs therefore reflects environmental changes or challenges to the fetus, and not directly that of cellular damage.

Cellular damage is much more likely to occur in the presence of both hypoxia and ischaemia locally at the cellular level (Schotz, 1953; Raichle, 1983; De Courten-Myers *et al.*, 1989), and this is not easily reflected by observable parameters such as fetal blood chemistry or the behaviour of the fetal heart. Cellular damage may result from other factors such as toxins and accumulation of waste products (Levine, 1959) and is reflected by the findings that factors other than hypoxia are implicated in adverse long-term outcomes. In retrospective reviews of children with permanent neurological deficits, it was shown that the majority of them had no demonstrable hypoxic episodes during labour (MacLennan *et al.*, 1999).

The relationship between these observable parameters and the final outcome for the fetus is therefore at best very approximate. This imprecise relationship has led to a call for the deletion of the term fetal distress, and a re-evaluation of the causes of adverse fetal outcome.

Nevertheless, intrapartum hypoxia remains a major preventable cause of long-term adverse outcome, and blood gas chemistry and fetal heart changes are the observable indicators of a fetus that may be in an hypoxic environment. These observations are therefore worthy of being made. The interpretation of these observations, however, needs to be made in the context of the overall clinical situation and within an understanding of the pathophysiology of hypoxia and cellular biology.

Fetal Physiological Response to Hypoxia

Intermediary metabolism

Acidic substances are the end-product of intermediary metabolism (Fig. 2.1). Carbohydrates are reduced to pyruvate through the anaerobic glycolytic pathway and pyruvate is metabolised by a series of dehydrogenase reactions in the Kreb cycle to produce carbon dioxide. During these reactions adenosine diphosphate (ADP) is converted to adenosine triphosphate (ATP) which provides the energy required in other vital metabolic processes.

During the dehydrogenase reaction, hydrogen is transferred to the hydrogen receptor nicotinamide adenine dinucleotide (NAD) to form NADH. This in turn reacts through a series of cytochrome reactions and combines with oxygen to produce water.

The end-products of metabolism are therefore water and carbon dioxide which combine to form carbonic acid.

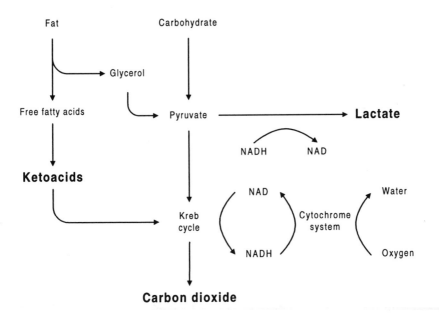

Fig. 2.1. Major pathways of intermediary metabolism.

In the presence of hypoxia, or if the cytochrome system fails for any reason, an alternative path is for NADH to pass hydrogen to pyruvate to produce lactate. This results in the accumulation of lactic acid.

If carbohydrate is deficient, fat is consumed. It breaks down into glycerol and free fatty acids. Glycerol enters the anaerobic glycolytic pathway but fatty acids are reduced to a variety of short-chain ketoacids, which are then metabolised via the Kreb cycle. These ketoacids are highly polar and acidic, and may be excreted in the urine and detected there as ketone bodies.

Fetal blood gas and pH

Excessive accumulation of carbon dioxide will result in respiratory acidosis (see Fig. 2.2), with a decrease in pH and increase in pCO_2. The accumulation of lactic acid or ketoacid will result in metabolic acidosis, where the decrease in pH is greater than can be accounted for by the increase in pCO_2.

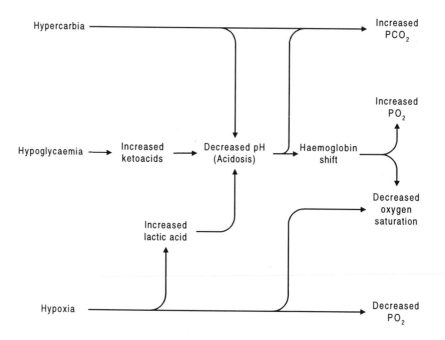

Fig. 2.2. Relationship between adverse metabolic events and blood gases.

Acidosis is caused by an increase in hydrogen ion concentration and this results in the displacement of oxygen from the haemoglobin molecule which in turn results in a reduction in oxygen saturation of haemoglobin and an increase in pO_2. Hypoxia therefore causes metabolic acidosis and results in a reduction of pH and oxygen saturation and an increase in pCO_2. Hypoxia has a variable effect on fetal blood pO_2, which may decrease because less oxygen is available but increase because of the effect of increased hydrogen ion concentration displacing oxygen from the haemoglobin.

Cardiac response

An increase in pCO_2 or hydrogen ion concentration stimulates chemo-receptors in the aortic arch and carotid bodies, and invokes a sympathetic response, and this in turn increases heart rate (see Fig. 2.3).

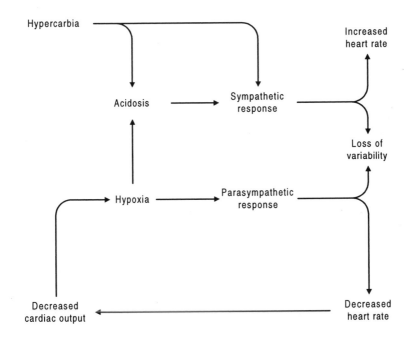

Fig. 2.3. Relationship between blood gases and cardiac function.

A decrease in pO_2 invokes a parasympathetic response, and produces a decrease in the heart rate. Under normal circumstances, sympathetic and parasympathetic discharges produce heart rate changes so that the fetal heart rate oscillates within a given range (variability). Exhaustive discharges from both sytems eventually reduce the abilities to respond and variability in heart rate is reduced.

Severe acidosis reduces cardiac contractility and this can reduce heart rate and a host of other ECG changes that are discussed in other parts of this book.

In addition to responses to pH and blood gas changes, heart rate and myocardial contractility are also affected by changes in the venous return, vagal response to head compression, arousal in response to touch and sound, sleep, and drugs. The many patterns of change in response to combinations of these effects are more effectively dealt with in a book on the CTG, and are beyond the scope of this chapter.

Changes in pH and blood gases, and changes in cardiac activity, in themselves have no direct effect on cells and hence long-term outcome. Where hypoxia and acidosis are sufficiently severe, cardiac failure or arrest occurs, and the fetus dies.

Cellular Effects of Hypoxia

Oxygen radicals

The biology of oxidative stress has been well described (Ceballos-Picot, 1997), and the following is a brief summary.

ATP is reduced to ADP during vital cellular chemical reactions and, in so doing, provides the necessary energy to fuel these reactions. ADP is converted to ATP during intermediary metabolism, completing the energy cycle.

A failure in metabolism results in an accumulation of ADP (Fig. 2.4), and this in turn is broken down into hypoxanthine. Some of this is further changed into uric acid and is eventually excreted.

Hypoxanthine also reacts directly with oxygen to produce free hydroxyl and oxygen radicals. These are ions with an extra electron attached and are

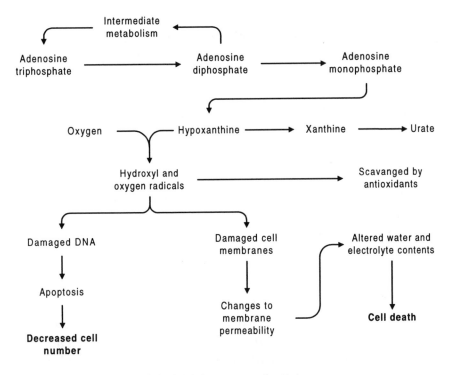

Fig. 2.4. Oxidative stress and cell damage.

chemically active. Cells with a good perfusion have an abundance of antioxidants and these scavenge free radicals as they are produced. Excessive amount of free radicals can result from excessive production or when insufficient antioxidants are available. These will chemically react with intracellular components, inducing cellular damage (Saugstad, 1996).

Membrane destruction

Free radicals react with lipoproteins, which are constituents of membranes, disrupting both their functions and structure. Damages to intracellular membranous structures disrupt metabolic processes and cause further production of free radicals.

Damage to cell membranes alters their permeability and the consequent influx of water changes the osmotic characteristics of the cytoplasm and causes the cell to swell. This as well as the influx of other ions also cause further metabolic disruption. Intracellular chemical changes, if severe, will result in cell death. Cell death may also occur when swelling causes the cell wall to rupture (Helliwell and Gutteridge, 1984; Koster *et al.*, 1986; Ward and Peters, 1995).

DNA damage

Free radicals may react with the chemical bonds responsible for retaining the shape of nucleoproteins. This results in the unfolding or fraying of the genetic strands. Such damage may trigger apoptosis and result in loss of the cell (Fawthorp *et al.*, 1991).

Cellular damage

Severe insults from free radicals may lead to cellular necrosis or rupture, and the resultant debris trigger an inflammatory response (Mongelli *et al.*, 1997; Rogers *et al.*, 1997; Wang *et al.*, 1997). The results may be observable neonatally and, depending on the structures involved, may present as encephalopathy, renal or cardiac failure, or necrotising enterocolitis (Low *et al.*, 1988; Low *et al.*, 1990; Socol *et al.*, 1994; Supnet *et al.*, 1994).

Less severe insults may not result in obvious necrosis and the associated inflammatory response, and these newborns may be indistinguishable from normal neonates. Apoptosis and cell loss, however, may result in intellectual deficits, motor disturbances or a reduction in the size of specific organs. These deficits may only be detectable much later on as developmental delays are observed.

Adverse long-term outcome

Adverse long-term outcome depends on cell death and cell loss, and these depend on oxygen radical damage. Such damage depends not only on metabolic failure, but also on reoxygenation aggravated by poor cellular perfusion.

Multiple factors of oxygen and reoxygenation, cardiac output and hypotension, local vascularity and vascular response, and preexisting health of the cells govern the extent of the damage. Many of these processes occur throughout pregnancy and after birth, and none of them is currently detectable clinically.

A Model for Fetal Distress

The current consensus seems to be that the term fetal distress should no longer be used as it confuses clinical signs and underlying pathology. The previous assumptions that hypoxia causes cellular damage and changes to pH, blood gas and cardiac functions are also recognised to be far too simplistic and cannot be supported by available evidence.

However, the concept that fetal hypoxia can have serious long-term consequences, that intrapartum fetal hypoxia is common, and that observable changes in fetal blood gas and cardiac function do reflect the existence of hypoxia, remains valid (see Fig. 2.5).

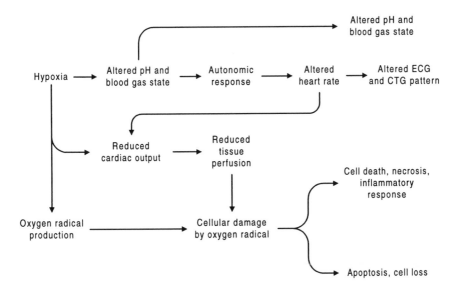

Fig. 2.5. Overall schema relating hypoxia, blood gases, fetal heart function and cell damage.

Chapter 3

RESEARCH MODELS AND PREDICTION

The Statistical Evaluation of Discrete Predictors

Researchers in obstetrics often use correlation or differences between observations of interest to define the underlying pathophysiology of fetal distress. When a statistically significant relationship exists between an observation with subsequent events, there is a potential to use that observation as a predictor (test). However, a statistically significant relationship merely defines that relationship to be closer than could be explained by random chance and the level of significance depends much on the sample size used. Other indices are therefore necessary for the evaluation of the utility of tests.

Once the existence of a relationship between a test and an outcome is assured, the performance of a test can be evaluated using observational data. As both test and outcome can either be positive or negative, four combinations result, as shown in Fig. 3.1. True positives (TP) are those where both test and outcome are positive, and true negatives (TN) are those where both are negative. False positives (FP) are those where the test is positive but the outcome negative, and vice versa for false negatives (FN). Indices of test performance can be derived from these combinations.

The sensitivity (SEN) of a test defines the probability that the test will be positive when the outcome is positive. The specificity (SPC) of a test measures the probability that the test will be negative if the outcome is negative. These two indices evaluate the quality of the test and are independent of the prevalence of the outcome. A highly sensitive test is

	Test Positive	Test negative
Outcome Positive	True Positive(TP)	False negative (FN)
Outcome Negative	False Positive (FP)	True Negative (TN)

Sensitivity = TP/(TP+FN)
Specificity = TN/(FP+TN)

Positive Diagnostic Value = TP/(TP+FP)
Negative Diagnostic Value = TN/(FN+TN)

Likelihood Ratio Positive Test = Sensitivity/(1-Specificity)
Likelihood Ratio Negative Test = (1-Sensitivity)/Specificity

Fig. 3.1. Combination of possible test and outcomes possible for one single test and one defined outcome. The values of these four combinations, true positive, false negative, false positive and true negative, can be used to determine statistical measurements, such as sensitivity and specificity, to allow assessment of test performance.

more useful for screening as few positive outcomes will be missed, while a highly specific test is more useful for making decisions to carry out risky interventions as more negative outcomes will be excluded.

The positive diagnostic value (PDV) of a test defines the probability an outcome will be positive when the test is positive. The negative diagnostic value (NDV) defines the probability an outcome will be negative when the test is negative. These two indices are dependent on the prevalence of the outcome in the population; the PDV increases and NDV decreases as the prevalence of the outcome increases. These indices are therefore evaluations of how useful a test is in a specific population.

The Youden index (SEN + SPC −1.0) summarises the sensitivity and specificity, while accuracy [(TP + TN)/Total] summarises positive and negative diagnostic values (Youden, 1950).

If one assumes that the occurrence of a positive test will lead to some form of therapeutic intervention but only a true positive results in benefit to the patient, then the inverse of the positive diagnostic value represents the intervention benefit ratio (IBR). With regard to the detection of fetal distress, this is represented by the number of inductions, other diagnostic tests, or operative deliveries required in order to reduce an incidence of a particular adverse outcome. For a test where the sensitivity and specificity are less than 1.0, the IBR increases exponentially as the prevalence of the morbidity decreases.

The Statistical Evaluation of Continuous Predictors

Many predictive tests are continuous measurements rather than discrete classifications. In order to convert this test to a discrete one, a threshold to decide when the test should be deemed positive is required. Any change to this threshold alters the number of true and false positives and negatives, and hence the performance of the test.

A number of conventions exist on how the threshold of a continuous predictor test should be determined after studying the reference data set. The most commonly used is a measurement two standard deviations from the mean of the normal (outcome negative) population, and using this to separate "normal" from "abnormal" values. Threshold can also be the value that produces the maximum Youden index or accuracy, in the belief that this will minimise error. Finally, a threshold can be the value at which the ratio of sensitivity and specificity correspond to their relative perceived importance.

A test can also be evaluated along the whole range of its measurements, independent of the threshold. This can be done by using the receiver operational characteristics (ROC) similar to that shown in Fig. 3.2. The relationship between sensitivity and specificity throughout its whole range can be plotted as a curved line and the area so defined represents the performance of the test. Henley and McNeil in 1982 produced statistical methods with which this area and its variance can be estimated from reference data. From these, the performance of difference tests can be statistically compared. De Long also produced a powerful method by which the ROC from two tests performed in the same population can be compared in a paired manner (Delong and Delong, 1988).

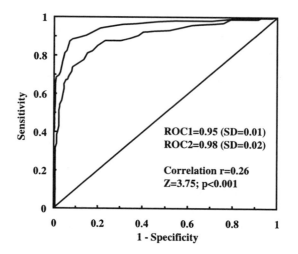

Fig. 3.2. An example of a receiver operating curve (ROC) showing values of sensitivity and 1-specificity. Individual and multiple tests may be compared to determine if they perform better than by pure chance by determining the area under each test curve.

The Validation of Predictive Tests by Observational Studies

The simplest method to validate a predictive test is to prospectively perform the test, observe the outcome, and see how the outcomes in the two groups compare. There are however a number of practical difficulties in carrying out this type of study.

Firstly, clinical events are highly variable and a test is performed in an instant within a long time frame of events. The information available and the clinical intervention that follow a test may therefore be highly variable and confound the results of any study.

Secondly, if a test is perceived to be useful, its result may lead to clinical intervention, which in turn prevents the predicted outcome, as shown in Fig. 3.3. The effective clinical use of a good test therefore statistically invalidates the relationship between the test and outcome. This is called the treatment paradox and accounts for the apparently disappointing results of many tests previously considered good after their introduction into clinical practice.

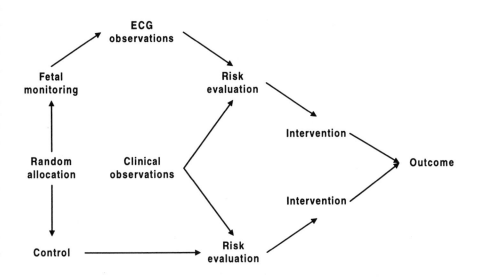

Fig. 3.3. Typical overview of a randomised controlled trial showing random allocation of subjects into a control and monitoring group, fetal monitoring in this case. The information available and the clinical intervention that follow a test are different in each arm of the trial, hence the reason and type of interventions may be different.

Lastly, a validating study to relate test and outcome therefore requires a clear definition of the population, a rigid management protocol, and the test results must be blinded to the clinicians who manage the patients.

The Validation of Predictive Tests by Clinical Trials

An alternative method of validating a predictive test is to conduct a clinical trial, randomly allocating different tests to groups, so that differences in outcome can be attributed to the tests. Randomised controlled trials have been an effective research technique across many disciplines, but its main use has been to clarify the effectiveness of different treatments or interventions. A trial of different predictive tests, therefore, has some differences in its structure.

As the clinician is not blinded to the tests, there are four resulting groups if two tests are compared. These are positive and negative outcomes predicted by Tests 1 and 2. From these, four sets of interventions and outcomes result, which are then combined according to which test is used. The results are therefore susceptible to confounding variables such as threshold values for different tests and how the clinical confidence in each of the test may affect subsequent management decisions.

The Inclusion of Both Intervention and Morbidity in a Clinical Trial of Predictive Tests

A test is only useful if the morbidity it predicts can be circumvented by appropriate intervention. A reduction in morbidity associated with its use is therefore invariably associated with an increase in interventions. The two related outcomes, intervention and morbidity, are therefore measured in the clinical evaluation of any predictive test. A change in intervention is however much more immediately obvious than that in morbidity.

The intervention benefit ratio (IBR) increases exponentially as the prevalence of morbidity decreases. Invariably, therefore, the increase in intervention exceeds the decline in morbidity when a predictive test is used (Mongelli *et al.*, 1997). In clinical decision-making, this discrepancy is accepted if a greater value is attached to the decrease in morbidity than the increase in intervention. In a clinical trial, however, the increase in intervention becomes much more marked than the decrease in morbidity.

Given that the IBR exists, the prevalence of intervention invariably exceeds that of morbidity, so the required power, and hence sample size, of an experiment to detect a change in morbidity is greater than that in intervention. An undersized study will likely lead to a conclusion that the use of a predictive test merely alters intervention but not morbidity.

The Hawthorne Effect

Conditions during a research study often differ from that of routine clinical care. Greater manpower may be available, more experienced personnel may be in charge and everyone is more careful. As a result, the outcome, particularly morbidity rate, improves. This is the Hawthorne effect. The planning of a study, if based on general clinical experience and without taking the Hawthorne effect into consideration, may seriously overestimate expected morbidity rate and prescribe a sample size smaller than the power requirement of the study.

Animal and Clinical Models of Study

Studies in fetal heart rate and ECG are based mainly on three models, namely, animal, antenatal and intrapartum studies.

The animal model is the only one where direct experimental manipulation of the fetus and its environment is possible, and so contributes to most of our understanding of the processes involved in fetal physiology. There are however a number of disadvantages in using this model. Some morphological and physiological differences do exist between experimental animals and humans, and how much these differences matter has yet to be fully explored. Some of the studies are acute experiments in sheep when the ewe is under general anaesthesia and tends to become acidotic, so it is not always clear how much the observations reflect artefacts introduced under experimental conditions. Finally, the experimental treatments applied are artificial, and although the results add understanding to the underlying physiological processes, they are not always generalisable to the clinical situation when the fetus is subjected to multiple interacting environmental factors.

The antenatal pregnant woman provides a good model for the study of heart rate. Both the mother and the baby are in a stable condition and there is no excessive signal interference from muscular or uterine activities. There is however no direct access to the fetus, so only a very weak signal is obtainable from the mother. Extensive signal averaging and enhancement are therefore necessary and the methods of doing these invariably change the signal. Another disadvantage is the difficulty of defining the outcome variable. The precise condition of the fetus is unknown, and a long time and many other events separate the study and delivery.

The fetus during labour has been extensively studied. Once the membranes have been ruptured, direct access to the baby is possible and a strong electrical signal is usually obtainable. The dynamic state of labour also provides many stimuli and much stress to the fetus, inducing changes that can be studied. Corroborative evidences of fetal distress, such as the passage of meconeum and changes in blood gases in the fetal blood, can be observed.

Signals can be obtained up to the time of birth, and correlation between signals and the condition of the baby at birth can also be evaluated. However, electrical signals obtained during labour are characterised by extensive noise, generated by muscular and uterine activities, and by the electrical equipment that surrounds the labouring woman. The signals are also altered by medications, such as oxytocin, analgesics and anaesthetic agents.

electrical activity through the heart causing the atria and ventricles of the heart to contract and relax.

The initiation and spread of the electrical activation in the heart under normal circumstances is controlled by the sino-atrial node. This node acts as the heart's pacemaker which, when fired, causes the spread of the electrical activation wave through the atrial myocardium. The atrioventricular node situated low in the right atrium picks up the electrical activity in the atrial myocardium and transmits this to the ventricular myocardium via the "bundle of His" and "Purkinje fibres" through which it then propagates. The transmission of the electrical activation in the atrial myocardium is different from that in the ventricular myocardium because, in the latter, the left and right bundles branch and the inferior divisions transmit the electrical signal received at the atrioventricular node almost simultaneously to all regions of the ventricles, whereas in the atrial myocardium, the effect of the electrical activation is analogous to that of a ripple in a pond after its surface has been disturbed by an object. Under normal conditions, the myocardium is a highly effective conductor of the electrical activity in all directions and its actual direction is highly dependent on the specific site of initiation. From this specific starting point, the predominant spread of the electrical activity will depend on where the greatest mass of myocardium is available.

The sino-atrial node is influenced by both the sympathetic and parasympathetic (vagal) nerves, the latter being more prevalent in the atrioventricular node, and of all the structures in the heart, it contains the greatest number of cells capable of "automaticity". These cells possess the ability to spontaneously produce a cardiac impulse. The sino-atrial node, therefore, controls the action of the heart as the cells in this node have the fastest automatic speed of response of all the fibres in the heart and the development of this ability occurs at the very early stages of embryonic development. Whilst other cells in the heart also possess the ability to act as pacemakers, their ability to do so is inhibited under normal conditions because the cells in the sino-atrial node are capable of producing cardiac impulses much faster and, hence in normal circumstances, they dominate all other possible pacemaker sites. The action of these cells, however, can be controlled as previously mentioned by the vagal and sympathetic nerves as well as chemically. Chemical agents, whether natural or externally introduced, such as circulating catecholamine levels, are capable of influencing the frequency at which these cells are capable of spontaneously generating cardiac impulses and hence heart beats. For example, increasing catecholamine levels causes an increase in heart rate.

The transmission of any electrical activity within the myocardium is dependent on any changes that occur at the cellular level. In a normal healthy myocardium, the cells are in a "polarised" state (i.e. a dipole, with equal numbers of positive and negative charges), that is to say, the outer surface of the cell membrane has an accumulation of positive charges which are in turn balanced by an equal number of electrons on its inner surface, as shown in Fig. 4.2(a). This remains the normal resting state of the cells until they are depolarised by the influence of an external stimulus which may be an artificial or a natural activation wave. As depolarisation occurs, the normal distribution of positive and negative charges is reversed so that the outer surface of the cell membrane becomes negatively charged and the inner surface positively charged. Initially, a small area of any given myocardial cell is induced to depolarise, as shown in Fig. 4.2(b), and as it does so, it causes other areas of the myocardial cell to spontaneously depolarise. As one cell becomes depolarised, its neighbouring cells are also induced to become depolarised producing a self-propagating wave through the myocardial cells, as demonstrated in Figs. 4.2(a)–4.2(c). The self-propagation of the depolarisation occurs because, at the junction of two cells, battery conditions apply. If one outer membrane is positively charged and its adjacent cell has a negatively-charged outer cell membrane, a local current will flow between cells, which in itself is enough to induce depolarisation in the adjacent cell and eventually in the whole myocardium.

The P wave and QRS complex can therefore be regarded as the resulting electrical activity produced by the propagation of the depolarisation wave through the atrial myocardial cells and ventricular myocardial cells. The recovery of the cells within the ventricular myocardium produces the T wave, which is therefore a repolarisation wave produced as the cells return to the original state of positively charged outer membrane. The recovery of atrial myocardial cells is masked by the electrical activity produced by the

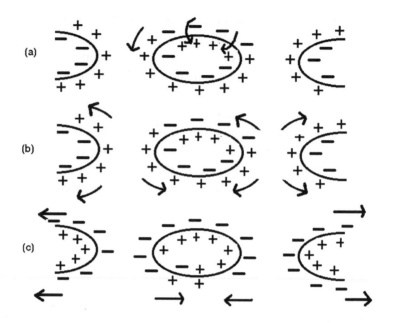

Fig. 4.2. Transmission of depolarisation effect from cell to neighbouring myocardial cells to generate a self-propagating waveform.

depolarisation taking place within the ventricles.

The shape of the individual components of a fetal electrocardiogram is dependent on the specific location of the electrodes which are being used to observe the electrical changes that are occurring with each cardiac cycle. If a single electrode, referenced to ground (unipolar), is placed on the surface of the heart and connected to a galvanometer, the needle of the instrument would be deflected upwards (positive) or downwards (negative) depending on whether the electrical impulse is seen to be moving towards or away from the electrode. In the normal electrocardiogram, the P wave is the profile of the electrical deflection which proceeds from the QRS complex and is usually smooth and round in shape. The QRS complex represents the spread of the electrical activation through the ventricles and is usually "spiky" in shape and often the largest deflection. The QRS complex is usually a combination of three components, the Q wave, R wave and S wave. The first positive wave associated with the electrical activation of the ventricles is always termed the R wave. Any negative going wave, either preceding or following the R wave, is termed the Q and the S wave, respectively. The last component, the T wave represents the electrical recovery of the ventricular myocardium. It usually follows the QRS complex and is usually a smooth broad wave separated in time from the QRS complex by what is termed the ST segment.

Acquisition of the Signal

Obtaining the signal — Electrodes

In adult cardiology, electrodes are positioned according to "Einthovens Triangle", allowing all aspects of the electrocardiogram components to be investigated since all known vectors of the signal can be predetermined. However, access to the fetus is not so convenient. Nearly all investigators prior to 1962, when Hon first introduced the general use of scalp electrodes, obtained their fetal electrocardiogram signals from electrodes positioned on the maternal abdomen. Due to the poor signal-to-noise ratio, these early studies (Southern, 1957; Larks, 1963) did not allow convincing and detailed evaluation of the electrocardiogram components. Smyth in 1953 described the first insertion of a silver wire into the amniotic sac and that enabled the fetal electrocardiogram obtained to be at least five times greater in amplitude compared to that of the background noise. Hon in 1963 described the use of his directly attached vaginal electrode, shown in Fig. 4.3, which was the precursor to the current modern scalp electrodes which are produced by a number of different manufacturers.

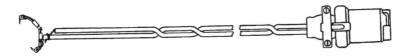

Fig. 4.3. Scalp clip electrode developed and used by Hon in his early work to obtain an adequate signal for calculation and recording of changes in the fetal heart rate during labour (reprinted with permission from Hon, 1963; copyright © Mosby, Inc.).

All direct scalp electrodes work on the same common principle. An electrode is directly attached to the presenting part of the fetus by penetrating the skin surface. The spiral electrode is screwed into the presenting part, whilst the Copeland clip works by skewering a piece of skin via the use of a spring-loaded clip. The electrode directly attached to the fetus is termed the "active electrode". A second electrode termed the "indifferent" electrode is used to make contact with the vaginal vault and cervix. A fetal electrocardiogram can therefore be obtained by determining the voltage difference between the active and indifferent electrodes when both are referenced to a common point (usually the maternal thigh).

Predominantly, most of the scalp electrodes designed were minor variants of that initially proposed by Hon. Goodwin and Unger in 1972 described a stainless steel pincer electrode that had been electroplated with silver. These scalp electrodes gave rise to signals ranging from 150–650 µV. Whilst not as large as the signals obtained from adults (typically several mV), they were considerably larger than those fetal electrocardiogram signals obtained by abdominal surface electrodes. Hon's work has led to three main types of scalp clips now being routinely used throughout the world, namely the single- and double-spiral, and the Copeland clip.

Whilst the scalp electrode remains the most commonly used method of obtaining an electrocardiogram, other techniques, such as using abdominal electrodes, surface electrodes, magnetocardiography and other non-invasive techniques, have been attempted in the antenatal and intrapartum periods (Wakai *et al.*, 1993; Mazzeo, 1994; Genevier *et al.*, 1995; Crowe *et al.*, 1996; Kwon and Shandas, 1996). These reported approaches remain experimental and have not as yet replaced the scalp electrode as the primary means by which an intrapartum fetal electrocardiogram is obtained for analysis.

Non-penetrating electrodes

As mentioned previously, scalp electrodes require penetration of the skin. There has therefore been a recent trend to the development and use of internal surface contract probes. These probes are often termed "non-invasive" which is not strictly correct since, whilst not being invasive to the fetus, they are still invasive to the mother. Four surface devices have been reported in the literature. Hoffmeyer and Spencer have both developed and reported on single-use probes which rely on suction to maintain surface contact (Hofmeyer, 1993; Bunn *et al.*, 1994; Gulmezoglu *et al.*, 1996; Spencer and Samson, 1998). Steer and coworkers developed a plastic probe with multiple sensors allowing not only maternal and fetal electrocardiograms to be obtained but also allowed observation of the amniotic fluid and intrauterine pressure (Antonucci *et al.*, 1997). The Steer probe was placed next to the fetus and relied on uterine pressure to maintain it in contact. Gardosi has reported on the development and use of a "balloon probe" which makes use of an inflatable bag which, when inflated, forms a wedge to keep the probe in apposition with the fetus (Gardosi, 1995). The eventual usefulness of any or all of these probes has yet to be demonstrated. Hoffmeyer's probe still has a failure rate of 30% and was only reported to have been used in 50 cases. Personal experience of the balloon probe and the Spencer probe, shown in Figs. 4.4 and 4.5, suggests that each is capable of providing a signal which at least is comparable in amplitude to that obtained from a Copeland scalp electrode.

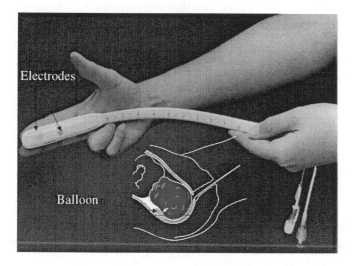

Fig. 4.4. Balloon electrode for use in the measurement of oxygen saturation and heart rate.

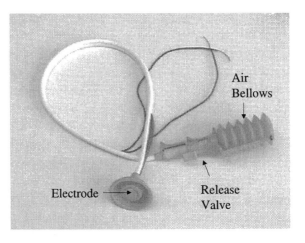

Fig. 4.5. Spencer electrode developed for non-invasive contact determination of the fetal electrocardiogram for rate calculation.

Electrode characteristics

One of the most important factors affecting the amplitude of signal obtained is the surface area of the actual clip that is in contact with fetal subcutaneous tissue. Early investigative work on the abdominal electrocardiogram made use of large surface electrodes (30 cm × 8.7 cm) in order to maximise the fetal electrocardiogram. The frequency characteristics of scalp electrodes in current use were first reported in 1990 by Westgate. The study described the frequency characteristics of the five most commonly used scalp electrodes and reported that the spiral electrode came closest to the ideal characteristics required for fetal electrocardiogram analysis. They demonstrated that the Copeland electrode gave rise to smaller signals, attenuated by approximately 50% when compared to the spiral. This can be linked to the actual total surface area of the Copeland clip embedded in subcutaneous tissue, the spirals being much greater than that of the Copeland. The frequency characteristics of the surface contact probes have not as yet been reported in the literature. The Nottingham group has compared the signal obtained by the Gardosi and Spencer probes with that of a spiral and Copeland clip. The amplitude of the signals obtained from the Gardosi and Spencer probes is comparable to that of a well-applied Copeland clip but not as large as that obtained by a well-applied spiral.

Electrode–tissue interface

The spiral and Copeland scalp electrodes are both manufactured from stainless steel, which is not the most effective conductor of electrons between the subcutaneous fetal tissue and any electrical circuit. Electrical current is carried by anions in the body and by electrons in the electrode and electronic hardware. An interface therefore exists between the tissue and the sensor as charges are transferred from one type of carrier to another. This resulting potential difference is amplified along with any biological signal being measured and is a potential source of signal distortion and time variation.

Different metals, namely brass, silver and gold, have been used to see if this potential difference can be minimised and hence provide a more stable electrode tissue interface, thereby reducing noise and baseline wander.

Vectors

As there is no direct means of access to the fetus, any study of the morphology of the fetal electrocardiogram during labour will be dependent on the degree of fixation of the scalp electrode to the scalp as well as its specific location. The degree of fixation will affect the amplitude of the signal obtained whilst its position will determine the vector of the fetal electrocardiogram. The standard scalp electrode is said to be sensitive to electrical voltage changes in the ZX axis. In studying morphological changes of the ST segment and the T wave, the ST analyser groups in Plymouth and Gothenburg suggested the use of the unipolar lead configuration in order to study changes in T wave, which they described as occurring predominantly along the Y axis. Lindecrantz *et al.* (1988) reported gross changes in the R/S ratio when using a bipolar scalp electrode in those labours where the head was seen to rotate and hence they suggested the use of a unipolar electrode configuration. Whilst these types of gross changes in morphology may be possible in extreme cases, routine study of the FECG in Nottingham, where the bipolar electrode arrangement has been used, has so far failed to produce a case where the orientation of the FECG is completely inverted or where the R/S ratio is significantly changed.

Signal Detection and Enhancement

Signal detection

The most recognisable component of the FECG is the QRS complex. All algorithms described so far in the literature try to detect this feature of the FECG. In the early investigative studies, the problem of detecting the fetal QRS complex was made more difficult by the presence of the maternal ECGs on the abdominal recordings. Before the fetal QRS complex could therefore be detected, the maternal signal must first be eliminated without distorting the QRS complex.

Several techniques have been described to perform the cancellation of the maternal ECG from abdominal signals. Hon and Hess in 1957 suggested that a maternal and an abdominal signal should be summed together using a differential amplifier, thereby eliminating the maternal ECG and leaving the fetal signal. The introduction of digital computers in the 1960 led to the design and development of more mathematically intense techniques to try and detect the most prominent feature of the ECG waveform, namely the R wave which acts as the primary reference point for subsequent waveform enhancement. The remainder of this section focuses on techniques which were used to detect the fetal R wave of the QRS complex from electrodes which were directly applied to the fetus.

QRS waveform detection algorithms can be divided into three broad categories. They can be thresholding algorithms, matching algorithms, syntactical algorithms or a combination.

The QRS detector, depending on its complexity, contains three principle components — a linear filter, a non-linear transformation and some decision logic to decide whether the R wave is present or not. The QRS detectors developed have become increasingly more sophisticated with the changes in software and hardware over the last three decades. The early R wave detection used a static threshold. This threshold could be lowered, raised or kept fixed depending on whether an automatic gain control module was used or not. Once the signal exceeded this threshold, an R wave was assumed to have been located. This technique was used in most early research as initial work focused on the changes in heart rate interval rather than changes in the waveform. Early signals were therefore heavily filtered in order to provide the detector with a stable baseline from which to detect departures. Friesen *et al.* in 1990 reported on the performance of several different forms of the QRS detector which had been described in the literature at that time.

More recent QRS detectors have employed software-matched filters which "ring" when a QRS complex is processed, as shown in Fig. 4.6. They are designed to match either the frequency characteristics or the shape of the QRS complex. Power spectral analysis of isolated ECG waveforms has shown that the QRS wave lies in the frequency range of 10–25 Hz. Bandpass filters can therefore be designed to target this range and, in so doing, identify the region of the signal where a QRS complex may exist. Band pass filters are therefore commonly used as the initial linear component of the detector. The resulting output signal from these filters is then mathematically transformed and integrated to provide an envelope in which to locate the R wave peak.

With the increasing power of signal processing chips, more complicated techniques, such as the use of neural networks and wavelet transformations, have been described in the literature to detect the QRS component of electrocardiograms (Xu *et al.*, 1993; Kadambe *et al.*, 1999).

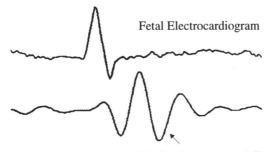

Fetal Electrocardiogram

Ringing from matched filter to indicate presence of QRS complex

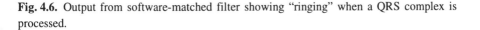

Fig. 4.6. Output from software-matched filter showing "ringing" when a QRS complex is processed.

Enhancement

Unlike the adult ECG, the FECG must first be enhanced before it can be analysed because of its poor signal-to-noise ratio. This enhancement has usually been in the form of a certain type of mathematical signal averaging on a fixed window of data about the R wave peak, which acts as the point of alignment (Smith and Kirk, 1986; Cano *et al.*, 1990; Escalano *et al.*, 1993). The size of window is set so that it is wide enough to include both the P and T wave complexes. Signal averaging allows a wanted repetitive signal, e.g. the FECG, to be extracted from the random background noise provided it is time aligned [time coherent enhanced averaging (TCEA)]. By using a fixed reference point on the waveform, repetitive signals are linearly added over a finite number of samples to produce an enhanced waveform whilst at the same time attenuating the noise. A number of techniques have been developed, ranging from simple group averaging to the use of digital low-pass filters. All these approaches are however reliant on the accurate detection algorithms capable of reliable location of a fiducial point on the waveform (Barabaro *et al.*, 1991).

The early work done by Hon and coworkers used a hardware computer, termed "CAT" (computer of averaged transients), which retrospectively calculated the group average of a selectable number of isolated ECG waveform complexes (Hon and Lee, 1963; 1964). This system was reliant on an external trigger to instruct the computer which waveforms were to be included. However, whilst group-averaging technique was used by many others at this time, its limitations were documented by Hon and Lee. They suggested that weighted- and running-weighted-averaging techniques would be preferable to group averaging in order to minimise the exclusion and attenuation of rapid short-term changes in the ECG waveform from the eventual enhanced waveform.

Rhyne described the adaptation of a weighted-averaging technique which gave the most recent FECG waveforms the most weighting and which permitted transient changes to be observed in the enhanced running-averaged waveform (Rhyne, 1968; 1970). Rhyne's averaging system was shown to be mathematically equivalent to a low-pass digital recursive filter and hence could be reproduced in a software form (Scott, 1970). Little use appears to have been made of TCEA in the analysis of the FECG waveform until the early 1980s when it was extensively used in automated computerised systems by Symonds and coworkers based at Nottingham University (UK) when studying changes of the fetal waveform and comparing these changes with

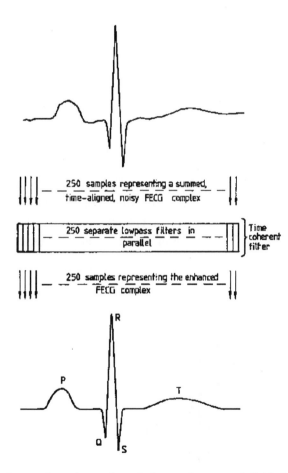

Fig. 4.7. Time-coherent enhanced averaging technique used to process individual digitised elements of the digitised raw waveform to produce a noise-free enhanced waveform.

subsequent metabolic status (Shield and Kirk, 1981; Jenkins *et al.*, 1986; Smith and Kirk, 1986). This was probably because of simultaneous improvements in the scalp electrode and fetal monitoring technology in the previous decade, allowing simpler technologies initially described by Southern (1957) to be still used.

The TCEA used by the Nottingham group employed a second-order low-pass Butterworth recursive digital filter for each individual digitised sample on the isolated waveform, as shown in Fig. 4.7. The effect of this filter on the waveform can be considered by looking at one single point on the waveform, the P wave peak. Successive values passed to the filter associated with this point will correspond to the P wave peak of successive complexes. Since changes in the FECG waveform occur relatively slowly, they are allowed to pass through the filter where randomly varying noise superimposed on the signal are attenuated. The relative weighting given to each complex can be determined by determining the impulse response of the filter, as shown in Fig. 4.8. This shows the behaviour of the enhancement filter used by Murray *et al.* (1986) when conducting both *in vivo* and *in vitro* analyses and validations of changes in human and sheep FECG waveform complexes. The degree of enhancement and responsiveness of the

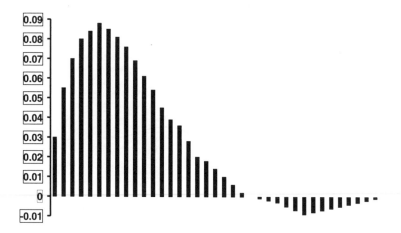

Fig. 4.8. Example of the relative weighting applied to each original complex. The weighting profile can be determined by deriving the impulse response of the filter.

enhanced waveform to dynamic changes in the underlying signal can therefore be changed by simply changing the relative cut-off frequency of the filter.

Other methods of signal enhancement include those of adaptive noise cancelling described by Widrow *et al.* in 1975 and Ferrara and Widrow (1982). This approach requires the use of a second reference signal which can be subtracted from the original signal in order to cancel out noise sources on the input (Thaler *et al.*, 1988; Crowe *et al.*, 1996.)

Pitfalls of using time-coherent enhanced averaging

Time-coherent enhanced averaging can result in some distortion of the waveform and hence a misrepresentation of the underlying biological signal if appropriate signal rejection techniques are not used or if there is poor R wave alignment, making any subsequent measurement unreliable and therefore limited in value (Bhargava, 1994). Some form of quality assurance must therefore be performed on each windowed segment of the FECG prior to its acceptance into the averaging process. This would include rejection of transient noise spikes, waveforms where the baseline drift, shown in Figs. 4.9(a)–4.9(c), is excessive and those waveforms where the hardware amplifiers have been saturated, producing a clipped waveform. Failure to exclude artefact of this type usually will result in signal attenuation of the final enhanced FECG and its eventual corruption. A number of simple rules which are listed below have been be used to reject windowed signals from the enhancement:

(i) Counting the number of digital samples of the FECG waveform in the windowed signal that are at the maximum value of the analogue-to-digital converter. This would exclude those waveforms which contain areas of the signal that have saturated the analogue-to-digital converter.

(ii) Checking to see if there is a large difference which could be defined between any two consecutive digital waveform sampling points. This will exclude sudden noise spikes.

(iii) Comparing the mean amplitude of a fixed number of points in the

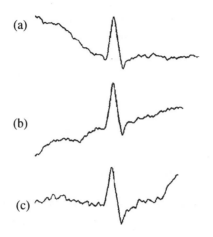

Fig. 4.9. Examples of waveform showing excessive baseline drift that would need to be rejected prior to performing time-coherent enhanced averaging in order to avoid corruption of the enhanced waveform.

windowed waveform at its beginning and end against a maximum-permitted difference. This will exclude waveforms of the type shown in Figs. 4.9(a) to (c) which all have large baseline shifts.

(iv) Summation of the point-by-point absolute difference between the existing enhanced waveform and new waveform to be incorporated. The sum obtained will give a measure of the overall noise present. Should this value exceed a set threshold, then waveforms can be rejected.

Although TCEA is a good method of enhancing repetitive waveforms, non-repetitive transient features are however removed by the averaging process. As a result, any arrhythmias which may occur in the FECG are attenuated as if they were just random noise components. The attenuation is even more pronounced when the arrhythmia contains FECG components whose time relationship with the QRS varies, an example being heart block. In such cases, the P wave of the enhanced waveform will seem to disappear.

Morphology and Time Measurement of the Enhanced Waveform

The availability of an enhanced FECG waveform has allowed objective assessment of changes in waveform morphology and time intervals to be investigated in a number of published clinical studies. Researchers studying dynamic changes have tried to automate this process because of the sheer volume of data that could be recorded for each waveform. Figure 4.10 shows the clinically accepted reference points with time intervals and amplitude measurements that could be recorded for each FECG complex. These reference points are adopted from definitions used in quantitative measurement of the adult ECG.

The definitions of the time intervals and morphological measurements of the FECG are shown in Table 4.1.

There are few references in the literature that have described methodology

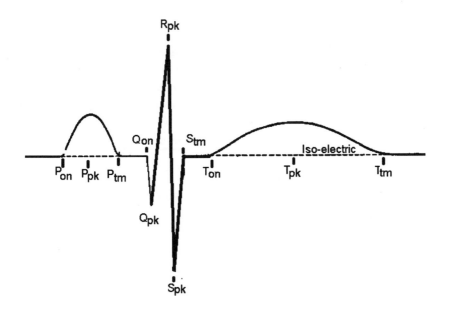

Fig. 4.10. Clinically accepted reference points with time intervals and amplitude measurements that could be recorded for each FECG complex. Most of these reference points are adopted from definitions used in quantitative measurement of the adult ECG.

for the automated morphological measurement of the FECG waveform, either antenatally or during delivery. The methodologies that do exist have relied on

Table 4.1 Definitions of temporal and morphological intervals in the fetal ECG.

Temporal

P wave duration	duration between onset and end of P wave.
PR interval	duration between P peak and R peak
RT interval.	duration between R peak and P peak.
QRS duration	duration between onset Q wave and end S wave
T wave duration	duration between onset and duration T wave

Morphological

P wave height	P wave amplitude
P wave area	area between the P wave and the isoelectric line
PR segment elevation	amplitude end of P wave to start of Q wave
Q wave height	Q wave amplitude
R wave height	R wave amplitude
S wave height	S wave amplitude
ST segment elevation	amplitude end of S wave to start of T wave
T wave height	T wave amplitude
T wave area	area between T wave and isoelectric line
R/S ratio	amplitude R wave divided by amplitude S wave

the use of idealised fixed templates and straight-line models or definitions which have been optimally matched to the FECG complex or waveform to be measured.

The straight-line model shown in Fig. 4.11, originally described by Marvel in 1978 and used by the Nottingham group, was used to determine the various FECG reference points shown in Fig. 4.10 (Marvel, 1978; 1980). In this model, a regression line was estimated for the rising and falling slopes as well as the isoelectric periods of the waveform, as illustrated in Fig. 4.12. The FECG reference points, such as the onset, peak and termination of individual complexes, can then be estimated by finding the point of intersection

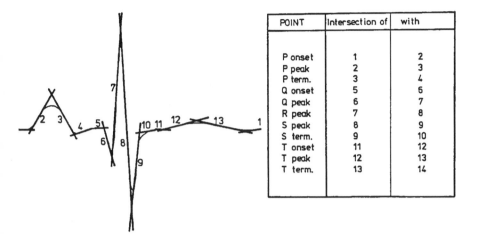

POINT	Intersection of	with
P onset	1	2
P peak	2	3
P term.	3	4
Q onset	5	6
Q peak	6	7
R peak	7	8
S peak	8	9
S term.	9	10
T onset	11	12
T peak	12	13
T term.	13	14

Fig. 4.11. The straight-line model used to determine the various waveform reference points on each enhanced waveform (from Smith, 1983).

between two fitted lines, as described in Fig. 4.11. In this way, the idealised straight-line template could be fitted to each enhanced waveform at defined regular intervals. Once the reference points have been determined, each waveform can then be characterised. FECG component amplitude measurements were expressed as a percentage of the R–S wave amplitude. This is done to make them independent of the original signal amplitude which is largely dependent on the degree of penetration of the scalp electrode into the fetal tissue. As in conventional cardiology, amplitude measurements were measured from the isoelectric line.

The Stan system, used by Westgate in clinical trials, differs from the Nottingham system in that no straight-line model was used (Lilja, 1980). This was because, initially, the only measurement made by this system was the height of the T wave, the T/QRS ratio. There were however differences between the estimation of T/QRS ratios between the Nottingham and Stan systems as identified by Skillern *et al.* in their *in vivo* and *in vitro* comparisons of the two systems (Skillern *et al.*, 1994). These differences can be explained by the different selections for the isoelectric level in the two systems. In the Nottingham system, the isoelectric period is then taken as the level of the waveform immediately prior to the P wave onset (pre-P wave) whereas the

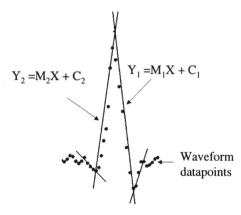

Fig. 4.12. Determination of the point of intersection using two regession lines, each representing one aspect of the waveform such as the rising and falling edges of the R wave.

Stan system has taken the level of the signal between the end of the P wave and the onset of the QRS complex, the PR segment. This difference becomes important only when the pre-P wave and PR segment are at differing levels, resulting in either an over- or underestimation of any amplitude measurement depending on the direction of the difference.

The remaining chapters of this book describe how the primary measurements obtained from processing of the obtained fetal electrocardiogram have been used either in clinical practice (R–R′ interval) or during research studies to determine the relationship between changes of the fetal electrocardiogram measurements and fetal condition.

Chapter 5

THE R–R′ INTERVAL
AND THE CARDIOTOCOGRAPH

The most commonly used parameter of the fetal ECG is the QRS complex and this is used in the calculation of the fetal heart rate from the R–R′ interval. It is not the intention of the authors that this book should concentrate on the monitoring of fetal heart rate as there are numerous excellent texts available on this subject and, moreover, this is a book about the FECG waveform. However, the book would be incomplete without some reference to the regulation of heart rate as calculated from the R–R′ interval.

Physiology of Fetal Heart Rate Regulation

The fetal heart rate varies throughout pregnancy and is regulated by a number of feedback mechanisms. The information taken from the fetal electrocardiogram for the calculation of fetal heart rate is derived from the time taken between successive R waves, which is then transposed mathematically into an expression of heart rate.

The initial embryological appearance of a single hollow ventricle occurs by five weeks of gestational age when a ventricular rhythm is established at 60–80 beats/minute. By the ninth week, the sino-auricular node has developed and the baseline heart rate is 175 beats/minute. It thereafter falls to a level between 110–150 beats/minute.

The rate at which the heart beats is regulated from a cortical and a subcortical level through the vasomotor centre in the medulla oblongata via the autonomic nervous system, and through the aortic and carotid baroreceptors and chemoreceptors.

Regulation by the Autonomic Nervous System

The heart has its own intrinsic rate as regulated by the sino-atrial (SA) node, a pacemaker in the atrium and the atrioventricular (A/V) node. The A/V node has the slowest inherent rhythm, as demonstrated in the bradycardia seen in the adult where there is a complete heart block.

Parasympathetic fibres can be identified in the fetal heart by the eighth week of gestation but full parasympathetic activity does not appear to be established until 32 weeks gestation.

The basal heart rate is influenced by a number of factors which include the vagal tone acting through the vagal and vasomotor centres and which acts both on the SA and AV nodes. Stimulation of vagal activity as initiated, for example, through head compression, results in bradycardia. The vagal tone exerts a major regulatory influence on the basal heart rate. On the other hand, increased sympathetic activity results in a slow rise in heart rate and an increase in myocardial contractility. Thus, baseline heart rate is not only determined by the balance of sympathetic and parasympathetic activities but is also influenced by cerebral cortical activity and by various hormonal factors, such as the release of norepinephrine and epinephrine from the adrenal medulla, thyroid hormones and insulin. Hypoxia and asphyxia induce a release of catecholamines into the circulation and thereby increase the fetal heart rate and heart rate variability (Dalton *et al.*, 1977; Pardi *et al.*, 1977).

Regulation by Baroreceptors and Chemoreceptors

The heart rate is also influenced by the activities of the baroreceptors in the aortic arch, which are stretch receptors and respond to rises and falls in blood pressure, and by chemoreceptors in the carotid sinus and in other central sites, which respond to changes in partial oxygen pressures.

Thus, stimulation of the baroreceptors by increased blood pressure results in a vagally mediated fall in heart rate and a prolongation of the R–R' interval.

Fetal Heart Rate Variability

The baseline fetal heart rate normally lies within a range of 110–150 beats per minute as classified by the International Federation of Obstetrics and Gynecology (FIGO, 1987). However, the rate varies continuously under normal physiological conditions. This pattern of variability in the heart rate reflects the regulatory impact of autoregulation by the autonomic nervous system, and it may also be affected by the sleep status of the fetus and by drugs that have an effect on the CNS.

Although both short-term and long-term variabilities can be assessed by the use of the R wave in the fetal ECG, pulsed Doppler ultrasound is only suitable to measure long-term variability.

Short-Term Variability

The phrase short-term variability describes the time intervals between successive R waves and is a sensitive mechanism for assessing the microfluctuations in the R–R' intervals. Ingemarsson *et al.* (1993), in their book on fetal heart rate monitoring, have summarised the issues related to short-term variability, which is a more sensitive tool for assessing baseline activity of the heart than heart rate.

However, its use in clinical practice is limited because it needs to be subject to computer analysis if it is to produce reliable information, and because nearly all antenatal monitoring is performed with the Doppler ultrasound which does not give accurate information at this level.

The microfluctuation in the time intervals between successive R waves is thought to be predominantly related to variable activity in the parasympathetic nervous system.

Long-Term Variability

Long-term variability refers to the fluctuations in heart rate over longer time intervals and therefore represents the macrofluctuations which are more readily used for clinical purposes. It may therefore be described in terms of oscillatory frequency or, more commonly, on the basis of amplitude or bandwidth. This can be assessed by detecting the heart beats by pulsed Doppler ultrasound or, most accurately, by the use of the fetal ECG and the R wave.

Long-term variability reflects the interplay between sympathetic and parasympathetic activity but there is a close correlation between short-term and long-term variabilities and when long-term variability is diminished, short-term variability is also reduced. Thus, the "silent" flat trace shows neither feature whereas both features are present in a recording of a normal fetal heart rate.

Hammacher's classification (1978) of long-term variability suggested the following scheme:

Silent pattern or absent variability < 5 bpm.
Reduced variability of 5–10 bpm or low variability.
Normal variability of 10–25 bpm.
Saltatory or increased variability > 25 bpm.

Following the pharmacological blockade of the autonomic nervous system in the mature fetus, it is still possible to see evidence of FHR variability, indicating that the autonomic nervous system is not the sole regulator of FHR variability. Indeed, influences from the cortical centres, diurnal rhythms, sleep patterns and respiration may all influence FHR variability (Dalton, 1977).

Sinusoidal patterns of the fetal heart rate are rare but, in this state, regular oscillations of heart rate can be seen with an amplitude that rarely exceeds 5–15 bpm, and where the oscillations occur only 2–5 times/minute with absent short-term variability and reactivity.

This pattern is thought to be associated with loss of neural control and tissue hypoxia in the fetal brain stem. The pattern has been seen to be associated with severe fetal anaemia and rhesus iso-immunisation.

Fetal Behavioural States

The fetus is subject to various states of consciousness and activity and these states are highly relevant to the baseline heart rate. These states are described as:

> State 1F — Absence of body movements and rapid eye movements — a sleep state.
> State 2F — Sleep state but with active rapid eye movements.
> State 3F — Intermediate state between fetal activity and fetal wakefulness.
> State 4F — Awake state — true wakefulness.

These states are not discernible until 36 weeks gestation. Episodes of inactivity are associated with low FHR variability and as these episodes rarely last longer than 40 minutes, an antenatal trace should be continued for a minimum of one hour before it is considered that FHR variability is pathologically reduced. Vibro-acoustic stimulation may wake the baby and produce a transient tachycardia.

High Fetal Heart Rate Variability

Fluctuations of the FHR with a bandwidth in excess of 25 bpm often occur in labour or following acoustic stimulation of the fetus. Animal data have shown that the saltatory pattern can be demonstrated by inducing acute episodes of hypoxia in primates and may therefore represent episodes of cord compression (Ikenoue, 1981).

Low Fetal Heart Rate Variability

Ingemarrson *et al.* (1993a) have summarised the loss of FHR variability defined as less than 5 bpm under the following headings:

(i) Prematurity — Tachycardia and reduced variability are common in labours before 34 weeks without associated acidosis.

(ii) Fetal tachycardia — A heart rate above 200 bpm is associated with low variability.

(iii) Drugs, such as pethidine, reduce FHR variability and these changes appear to be associated with a change in the fetal behavioural state and, presumably, may be mediated through the CNS. Similar effects may be produced by beta-blockers.

(iv) General anaesthesia.

(v) Fetal malformations — These malformations of both the CNS and fetal heart are associated with reduced variability.

(vi) Hypoxia — This is clinically the most important factor associated with low heart rate variability. Cerebral damage during the antepartum period resulting from prolonged hypoxia is often associated with a loss of fetal movements and absent FHR variability. Low variability and persistent tachycardia are associated with fetal acidosis in about half of these cases. However, low variability can be seen for many hours in labour without being associated with fetal acidosis.

Accelerations and Decelerations of the Fetal Heart Rate

Accelerations

Ingemarrson *et al.* (1993a) have defined accelerations as a transient increase in fetal heart rate of at least 15 bpm and lasting at least 15 seconds, with the exception of cases where the baseline variability is low and where an amplitude of 10 bpm may be considered to be an acceleration.

Accelerations reflect dominance of sympathetic activation over para-sympathetic regulation and are associated with fetal movements. The presence of accelerations, therefore, is an important indicator of fetal well-being whether in the antenatal period or during labour. Antepartum accelerations detected by pulsed Doppler ultrasound are usually associated with fetal movements and give rise to what is known as a reactive CTG.

Repeated fetal movements over a sustained time interval may give rise to what appears to be an apparent baseline tachycardia. If the baseline returns to normal during or following contractions which restrict fetal movements, then the appearance may be one of late decelerations. On the other hand, accelerations may appear during contractions in association with fetal movements.

The absence of accelerations and the depression of baseline variability often coexist and, in this case, may be a sign of fetal hypoxaemia. Late decelerations that interrupt accelerations may indicate compensation of a healthy fetus for cord compression. Accelerations may occur after direct fetal stimulation by palpation, scalp blood sampling or vibro-acoustic stimulation.

In summary, fetal heart rate accelerations which can be detected by ultrasound or the fetal ECG indicate sympathetic nervous system activity and good fetal health. Conversely, the absence of accelerations is not invariably associated with fetal hypoxaemia and must be absent for at least one hour to have any clinical significance.

Decelerations

Decelerations, unlike accelerations, are generally pathological and are produced either by the central nervous system or by baroreceptor reflex activity. There is an extensive literature on the subject of decelerations and their interpretations in clinical practice. Furthermore, the lack of specificity of FHR monitoring has now given rise to many questions as to its value in clinical practice, and to the reliability and consistency in the interpretation of FHR patterns.

Since the early identification of the significance of heart rate decelerations, various classifications have been proposed. Caldeyro-Barcia in 1966 first described Type 1 and Type 2 dips, but the most widely used classification was published by Hon in 1968.

Early decelerations

The definition of decelerations during labour depends on the demonstration of uterine contractions. These decelerations begin early in the uterine contractions and have their nadir at the peak of the contractions and return to the previous baseline before the end of the contraction.

The heart rate does not usually fall below 100 beats/minute. These decelerations are believed to be due to head compression during uterine contractions resulting in raised intracranial pressure and vagally induced bradycardia. These patterns are rarely associated with fetal hypoxaemia or fetal acidosis.

Late decelerations

The onset of late decelerations occurs after the uterine contraction has become established, and the nadir of the heart rate occurs at least 15 seconds after the peak of the contraction wave so that recovery of the fetal heart rate occurs well after completion of the uterine contraction. The early studies of Beard *et al.* (1971) showed that a pattern of baseline tachycardia associated with late decelerations was the most significant indicator of fetal acidosis and had the worst clinical prognosis.

Variable decelerations

These decelerations vary in duration and intensity, and in their timing in relation to uterine contractions. The decelerations are thought to be the result of cord compression resulting in a reduced return of blood to the right atrium which may originally lead to a sympathetic stimulation and transient tachycardia, followed by a deceleration that is probably mediated through baroreceptor and chemoreceptor reflexes.

This type of deceleration occurs in approximately 25–30% of all labours. However, the significance appears to vary according to the pattern of decelerations. Krebs *et al.* in 1983 described pure variable decelerations which show an initial acceleration followed by a rapid deceleration, and then by a rapid return to the baseline FHR and a secondary acceleration.

A typical variable decelerations are characterised by a number of features, including loss of initial and secondary accelerations, slow return to the baseline and biphasic decelerations. These findings are associated with a lower cord blood pH than in pure decelerations. Shields and Shifrin (1988) have described a pattern of variable decelerations where a mild variable deceleration with overshoot in combination with a normal baseline frequency and persistently absent variability is associated with post-maturity, meconium staining, intrauterine growth retardation and neonatal seizures. These authors found that this pattern was identified in one third of 75 cases with cerebral palsy.

Interpretation of the CTG

It is not the intention of this book to discuss in depth the status of fetal heart rate monitoring as the main purpose is to present available data on the fetal electrocardiogram. However, as previously stated, the distance between consecutive R waves forms the basis for fetal heart rate measurement and some reference will be made about the present difficulties in the interpretation of the FHR.

The "ground rules" for fetal monitoring were established between 1960 and 1980, and the decade of the 1990s has largely seen the escalation of litigation based on the CTG which has led to a re-evaluation of the usefulness of the technique. Counting the heart rate both antenatally and in the intrapartum period was introduced to prevent intrapartum stillbirths, and although later studies have tended to suggest that it fails in this objective, early studies showed a substantial fall in the number of intrapartum stillbirths in relation to the number of antepartum deaths. However, the expectation that the technique would reduce the incidence of cerebral palsy and other forms of brain damage was an extrapolation that was likely to be confounded by the general issues of causation in relation to cerebral palsy. If one works on the assumption that cerebral palsy occurs in two or three cases/1000 deliveries, then a large data base is necessary to prove a reduction in the incidence as a consequence of any interventional technique. Accepting the studies of Blair and Stanley (1988) showing that intrapartum asphyxia is a rare cause of cerebral palsy and probably accounts for only 10–15% of cases, then we are talking about 1:5000 deliveries as a potentially preventable case of intra-partum damage and thus proving benefit becomes extremely difficult. The time gap between death and damage is small and hence the relatively small number of cases of cerebral palsy arising from intrapartum hypoxia.

The situation is further complicated by the limitations of using only one variable as a method of assessment and by the notorious deficiencies of clinicians in assessing accurately the CTGs. Lotgering and coworkers in 1982 studied the inter- and intra-observer variabilities in five obstetricians who were each given 100 antepartum recordings to interpret. One observer was given the same set of recordings on three separate occasions with intervals of at least four weeks. The inter-observer agreement was found to be low for all variables whereas the intra-observer variation generally showed consistent and good agreement for all variables. Nielsen and coworkers (1987) gave four experienced obstetricians 50 intrapartum CTGs which were assessed twice with a two-month interval. The observers had to say if the fetus was or would be compromised as judged by a one-minute Apgar score below 7, an umbilical pH < 7.13 or a need for primary resuscitation. Only 22% of the CTGs were assessed in the same way on the second reading by all of the obstetricians. In 1991, Donker reported a large study involving 22 experts from 10 EC countries with 17 selected CTGs. He asked them to segment and classify the CTGs. In a detailed and complex study, the results showed that the kappa group agreement values for accelerations and decelerations were good but agreement was generally poor for both the baseline variability and the types of decelerations.

Essentially, the only way that the variability of interpretation would likely be overcome would be to utilise computer analysis. This subject is reviewed in a later chapter.

Computerised Assessment of the RR Interval — New Definitions

Algorithms and modalities for the direct and indirect assessments of the heart rate (RR interval) are currently being developed and assessed in order to overcome the inconsistencies in interpretation by clinicians described earlier in this chapter. These algorithms have tried to mathematically represent the concepts and parameters that clinicians are trying to identify or measure when interpreting changes in the fetal heart rate. There have been publications of a number of algorithms or mathematical formulae which have tried to measure or determine the baseline, the type and shape of the deceleration and the type and extent of any variability which may be present. The original definitions published in the 1960s by Hon and coworkers, and subsequently revised, were eventually formalised to form the FIGO guidelines for the interpretation of the heart rate (FIGO, 1987). A closer examination of these guidelines would show that most are unsuitable for computerised assessment. This is demonstrated by the FIGO definition on how a baseline rate should be determined. The baseline as defined by FIGO is the mean once all accelerative and decelerative episodes have been removed. However, accelerative and decelerative periods are defined as departures from the baseline. Such circular definitions are therefore unsuitable for computerised assessment and hence a new set of research guidelines for the interpretation of the RR interval changes were published in 1997 by a working party of the National Institute of Child Health (NICH). The definitions listed in these guidelines were developed not only to aid visual interpretation but also to make them adaptable to computerised assessment. In some instances, these definitions will differ from those quoted earlier in this chapter.

Baseline

The most important definition described in the NICH guidelines was that of the baseline as without it, decelerations and accelerations cannot be detected. This was defined as the mean heart rate to the nearest five beats of a ten-minute segment after excluding periodic episodes, periods of marked variability or segments of the heart rate that differ by more than 25 bpm with the mean being calculated from a minimum of two minutes of data. This definition is however still circular and computerised algorithms that obtain their baselines in this way must perform repeated multiple passes through the available heart rate data in a manner similar to that described by Coppens and Dawes. The relative merits of performing multiple passes as opposed to a single pass are discussed later.

Baseline variability

These have been categorised as fluctuations about the baseline and are quantified as the peak to trough amplitude. Variability is then classified according to this amplitude as listed below:

Absent — Range unmeasurable, i.e. amplitude = 0
Minimal — 0 < amplitude range < = 5 bpm
Moderate — 5 < amplitude range < = 25 bpm
Marked — Amplitude > 25 bpm

Accelerative episodes — Accelerations

This definition is similar to that described earlier in this chapter (increase above the baseline > 15 bpm for more than 15 seconds) with the peak occurring within 30 seconds of the initial departure). An additional criterion is that the peak should occur within 30 seconds of the onset of the acceleration. If the acceleration lasts for more than two minutes but less than ten minutes, it is defined as being prolonged, otherwise, it should be regarded as a change in the baseline.

Decelerative episodes — Decelerations

The guidelines provide definitions for both classifying the type of deceleration and whether they are recurrent or not. In general, all decelerations can be quantified according to the depth of the nadir below the most recently calculated baseline and the time taken from their initial departure to their eventual return to the baseline.

Late decelerations are defined as decelerations that take more than 30 seconds to reach their nadir, which are associated with uterine contractions, and where the nadir of the deceleration occurs after the peak of the contraction.

Early decelerations are defined as decelerations that take more than 30 seconds to reach their nadir, which are associated with uterine contractions, and where the nadir of the deceleration and the peak occur simultaneously.

Variable decelerations are defined as decelerations that take less than 30 seconds to reach their nadir. In addition, the nadir must be at least 15 bpm below the baseline and must last for at least 15 seconds but less than two minutes.

A deceleration is said to be prolonged if the nadir is at least 15 bpm below the existing baseline and the duration of which is longer than two minutes but less than ten minutes. If a decelerative period lasts for longer than ten minutes, then it is a change in the baseline.

Computerised Systems for the Interpretation of Antepartum Fetal Heart Rate

The most widely used computerised antenatal heart rate analysis system is the Oxford Sonicaid System 8000 which was developed by Dawes and coworkers (Dawes *et al.*, 1991). This system and its variants have been widely reported and used to evaluate the antenatal fetal heart rate and its changes from the second trimester until delivery (Pello *et al.*, 1991; Dawes, 1999). Other antenatal systems used in analysing antenatal heart rate are the PORTO system (Bernades *et al.*, 1991; Bernades *et al.*, 1997), the Nottingham system (Vindla *et al.*, 1997) and that developed by van Geijn and his coworkers in Holland (Mantel *et al.*, 1990). The latter two systems are being primarily developed to study fetal behavioural state changes. Antenatal systems have the advantage of not being restricted in the complexity of the algorithms developed for extraction of the variables used to characterise the heart rate changes. This is because, firstly, the records are usually of a short defined period and, secondly, the computerised system is not required to give an immediate continuous interpretation for the purposes of clinical management. This lack of restriction has allowed algorithms to be used, which have employed a multi-pass approach to repeatedly analyse the primary heart rate and interval data as shown in Fig. 5.1.

The System 8000 and the Dutch system employed digital filtering techniques in order to isolate the baseline from transient departures by regarding fetal heart rate measurement as a signal composed of multiple frequency components, each representing a different aspect or parameter of interest. Figure 5.2 can be used to conceptually model changes in the fetal heart rate. Firstly, there are the low-frequency signal components which can be used to represent the baseline. Secondly, there are the medium-frequency components used to represent episodic departures, such as accelerations and decelerations and lastly, there are the high-frequency components which can

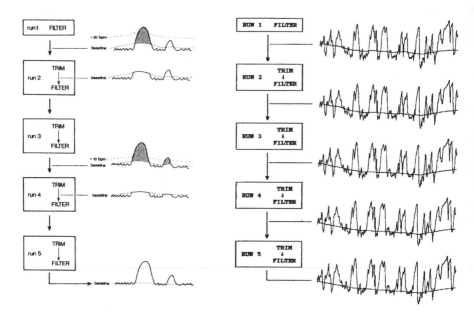

Fig. 5.1. Example of an algorithm using a repeated multi-pass technique to determine the fetal heart rate components of data collected from antenatal recordings (reprinted with permission from Mantel *et al.*, 1990; copyright © Elsevier Science).

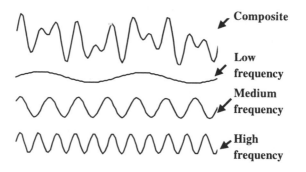

Fig. 5.2. Schematic representation of the fetal heart rate signal and its constituent components. A large number of fetal heart beats can be decomposed into their defined frequency components representing baseline (low frequency), variability (high frequency), accelerations and decelerations (medium frequency).

be used to measure variability. Each of these components has different periodicity and amplitude and, when summated, form the fetal heart rate.

Computerised Systems for the Interpretation of Intrapartum Fetal Heart Rate

The interpretation of intrapartum fetal heart rate is more difficult due to the greater variation of the fetal heart rate in labour. Intrapartum systems are also required to interpret in real time to be clinically useful, as events occur much more rapidly. The system is therefore more reliant on precise and appropriate electronic hardware while software algorithms must perform within the time constraints of frequent data input. Intrapartum systems should therefore be able to determine the baseline, variability, accelerations and decelerations, and process these into diagnoses between two successive samples of heart rate data. A number of computerised systems which have attempted to analyse the fetal heart rate in labour have been developed (Arduini *et al.*, 1994; Keith *et al.*, 1995; Todros *et al.*, 1996; Green, 1996; Bernades, 1998). The remainder of this section briefly describes the approach used by some of the algorithms that have been employed to extract features such as the baseline and variability in these systems.

Computerised estimation of baseline

The baseline is described in the guidelines as "the mean level of the fetal heart rate when this is stable, accelerations and decelerations being absent, determined over a period of ten minutes and expressed in beats/min" (FIGO, 1987). Whilst this appears a relatively simple definition, there are several ways by which the mean level may be calculated (Dalton and Dawson, 1984; Abduljabbar *et al.*, 1993; Chung *et al.*, 1995; Bernades *et al.*, 1996; Mongelli *et al.*, 1997).

One method of determining the baseline is the calculation of the arithmetic mean over a defined period of time as described by Chung *et al.* in 1995. This algorithm first calculated the mean of FHR values over a six-minute period which had been pre-processed by a low-pass filter to remove the effects of beat-to-beat variability. This algorithm, whilst working well on retrospective data, was found to be unresponsive to sudden large deviations in the baseline.

A second method which may be adopted is modified from the multiple-pass approach used by Dawes in System 8000. Firstly this determines the mode for a defined time period (ten minutes), which is used as a gate to exclude accelerations and decelerations. The remaining data is then repeatedly subjected to a low-pass filter until a stable baseline value is obtained. This method does require several passes of the data thus requiring additional computer processing time. It is also highly dependent on an adequate initial modal value being selected and is unstable during periods of high variation when a distinct modal value cannot be determined.

A third method is a combination of the mode and the arithmetic mean as described by Mongelli *et al.*, (1997). Firstly, the modal range, and not the modal value for a segment of FHR, is determined. The baseline can then be calculated as the arithmetic mean of this modal range. With the increased processing power and memory size now available, it is possible to create large storage arrays to determine the modal range. This technique offers several advantages over the previously described methods. Firstly, data may be analysed in a single pass. Secondly, the algorithm is more stable to small fluctuations and yet responsive to sudden changes. Thirdly, baseline values can be updated continuously with each new data point. When tested against a group of clinical experts, close agreements can be shown between the output of this method and clinical estimations of baseline values.

Computerised estimation of variability

A number of mathematical formulae and techniques have been used to quantify variability of fetal heart rate tracings, some of which are listed in Table 5.1. These methods can be summarised as belonging to one of five categories which are as follows:- modification of the mean, variation of the standard deviation, sorting and selection, slope changes and spectral analysis.

Table 5.1. Some of the published mathematical techniques and indices that have been used to quantify short- and long-term fetal heart rate variability.

Variability Index Authors	Index Category	Variability Measured STV	LTV
De Haan *et al.* (1971)	III	Yes	Yes
Tarlo *et al.* (1971)	II	Yes	
Yeh *et al.* (1973)	II	Yes	
Wade *et al.* (1976)	I	Yes	
Dalton *et al.* (1977)	I and II	Yes	Yes
Modanlou *et al.* (1977)	I	Yes	
Organ *et al.* (1978)	I and II	Yes	Yes
Young *et al.* (1978)	III	Yes	
Huey *et al.* (1979)	IV	Yes	Yes
van Geign *et al.* (1980)	III	Yes	
Zugaib *et al.* (1980)	I	Yes	Yes
Aboud and Sadeh (1990)	V	Yes	Yes

Index Category
    I. Indices using a modification of the mean
    II. Indices using a variation of the standard deviation
    III. Indices which are based on a sorting and selection approach
    IV. Indices which compute slope changes
    V. Power spectrum analysis

Variability Measured
    STV = Short-term variability
    LTV = Long-term variability

One of the simplest methods used was the determination of the standard deviation for a given segment of the trace (Yeh *et al.*, 1973; Organ *et al.*, 1978; Chung *et al.*, 1995; Vindla *et al.*, 1997). This method, however, will only work well when areas of the trace containing accelerations and decelerations have been excluded.

Another method is the use of a digital high-pass filter to isolate the high frequency component. Once this is done, variability can be quantified using

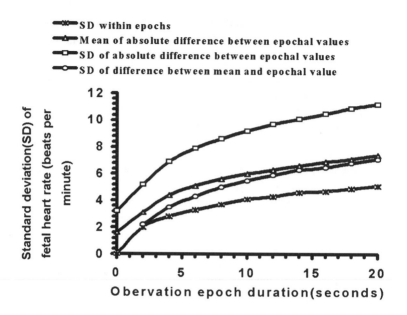

Fig. 5.3. Graphical illustration showing the effect of increasing sampling interval on the assessment of variability (reprinted with permission from Wilcox *et al.*, 1997; copyright © American College of Obstetricians and Gynecologists).

either the absolute range around the mode or the standard deviation over a defined period of time.

Variability may also be estimated by using the absolute differences between successive digitised samples of fetal heart rate values. These differences may then be analysed in a similar fashion as that of the digital high-pass filter to obtain an estimation of variability. The sampling interval, the time between two successive samples, should be considered when estimating variability from heart rate samples taken at regular intervals (Wilcox *et al.*, 1997). Figure 5.3 shows the effect of increasing sampling interval on the assessment of variability when compared to variability derived from all available data. The inappropriate choice of sampling interval will result in an under- or over-estimation of variability.

Mathematically, more intense techniques have also been applied in an attempt to try to quantify variability both in animal experiments and in human subjects (Cerutti *et al.*, 1989; Ferrazzi *et al.*, 1989; Lindecrantz *et al.*, 1993; Groome *et al.*, 1994). These have included the use of power spectrum and frequency determination, chaos and fractals (Shono *et al.*, 1991; di Renzo *et al.*, 1996) in order to characterise and determine patterns which exist in the variability data, such as breathing activity and mouthing (Natale *et al.*, 1988; van Woerden, 1990), autonomic state (Karin *et al.*, 1993), and fetal well-being (Sibony *et al.*, 1994)

The ability of mathematical indices to represent variability as defined by the clinicians has rarely been tested, either using simulated data or actual fetal heart rates. Studies that did compare relative performance against a simulated signal or using human and animal models are published by Parer *et al.* (1985), Kubo *et al.* (1987) and Knopf *et al.* (1991). The Parer study made use of sine waves of varying frequencies and amplitudes, and alternating beats of increasing intervals to test the ability of 22 different indices to measure changes in short and long-term variabilities in their stimulated signals. They concluded that indices which quantified short-term changes in variability were able to track and follow interval changes in their simulated signals. However, only one of the published indices (Huey *et al.*, 1979) at the time of the study could accurately quantify long-term variability. In the Knopf study, three observers' subjective assessments of variability were compared with that of the mathematical indices. Knopf and his colleagues concluded that the mathematical indices of short-term variability compared closely to its subjective evaluation of being present or absent. The long-term variability of indices also increased progressively with the observers' evaluations of increasing variability, and that both short- and long-term indices were able to quantitate what they clinically regarded as fetal heart rate variability.

Computerised identification of decelerations

Several computerised algorithms for the detection and classification of decelerations have been described in the literature. These have used either rule-based algorithms, neural networks or a combination of both modalities in their attempts to reliably detect decelerations. Maeda in 1990 extensively used the slope of the rising and falling edge of decelerations along with amplitude information to decide if departures below the baseline were decelerations. Keith in 1994 attempted to use a back propagation neural network to firstly identify the deceleration and then classify it. This did not however prove successful due to the variety of possible shapes and durations of decelerations. Their paper did however suggest that features of decelerations rather than the heart rate data itself should be processed in order to obtain a consistent detection rate.

An alternative approach of describing decelerations would be to quantify the time of the deceleration as well as their number and area, as originally described by Tipton and Shelley as early as 1971. The area of the deceleration, which represents the number of heart beats lost from the baseline can then be calculated. Any calculated area may also then be subdivided according to its relationship to that of the contraction peak. The study conducted by Tipton was hampered by having to make and weigh paper cut-outs equal in size to the deceleration in order to quantify them. However, with the advent of modern signal processing and direct access to the fetal heart rate measurements from the fetal monitor, deceleration areas, onsets, nadirs and ends can now be determined.

Chapter 6

THE INTERVALS AND MORPHOLOGY
OF THE FETAL ECG

A recording of the fetal electrocardiogram produces a vast amount of data which, if appropriately processed, can open a window on the performance of the fetal heart and act as a barometer for biochemical changes in the fetus. The fundamental difficulties that have limited the use of fetal electrocardiography as a tool for the assessment of fetal welfare are, firstly, the need to separate the signal from the fetal heart from a morass of background noises and secondly, the whole question of whether relationships between the time intervals and fetal acid–base balance are linear or whether because of the innate ability of the fetus to buffer changes induced by fetal hypoxia, the relationship is non-linear and only becomes revealing *in extremis*.

Since the very first description by Cremer in 1906 using a combination of vaginal and abdominal electrodes and a string galvanometer, investigators have struggled with the development of systems that can both isolate and measure subtle changes in the electrical activity of the fetal heart. Vast quantities of data are regularly discarded from the fetal ECG signal where commonly only the R–R' interval is utilised, but advances in signal processing now make it possible to build up a detailed real-time model of the electrical activity of the fetal heart without using excessively invasive techniques and our intention in reviewing the current state of fetal electrocardiography is to draw attention to the potential value of this technology.

The fetal electrocardiogram is essentially a map of the action potentials generated throughout the cardiac cycle. As discussed in Chapter 4, the cycle starts with the depolarisation of the sino-atrial node as a result of membrane potentials of pacemaker cells and this is associated with a dramatic influx of Na^+ and an efflux of K^+ ions. At the same time, an influx of Ca^{++} results in upstroke of the action potential in the SA node. Subsequently, the upstroke of the action potential in the atrioventricular node depends on both slow Ca^{++} channels and on the relatively fast oxygen insensitive Na^+ channels.

The PR interval reflects the conduction time in the AV node and the QRS complex represents ventricular depolarisation whilst atrial repolarisation is buried within the QRS complex. The ST segment and T wave reflect ventricular repolarisation.

Analysis of the FECG

The real difficulty about the analysis of the FECG is that the signal is often distorted by electrical noise, in particular 50 Hz interference, but also extraneous noise from other maternal and fetal sources. These issues have been addressed in detail in Chapter 4 but are rehearsed briefly here in the context of their importance to this chapter.

Part of this noise and the need for signal modification can be minimised by the use of appropriate scalp electrodes. The single spiral electrodes manufactured by Corometrics Medical Systems, USA, have a high signal amplitude and a good frequency response and low signal-to-noise ratio (Westgate *et al.*, 1990), but the Copeland electrode has also been shown to have characteristics that are adequate for the measurement of the time intervals of the FECG.

Development of an Analyser of the FECG

The development of a system that could provide real-time analysis has been the subject of continuing research at the Department of Electrical and Electronic Engineering at the University of Nottingham, and reference has already been made in previous chapters to the nature of this work.

Nevertheless, as much of the information presented in this chapter was derived from the Nottingham system, a brief summary of this work is needed in the context of many of the studies presented here. The work is otherwise dealt with in detail in Chapter 4.

Signal isolation and identification are achieved by digitisation of the analogue FECG and the use of matched filters to recognise the QRS complex by comparison of frequency spectrum characteristics. By using a time-coherent approach, an averaged waveform is developed around the R wave peak that thereby becomes the fixed point around which the raw signals are superimposed. The averaged waveform obtained from this process of the time-coherent enhanced averaging regime has removed non-repetitive features such as electrical noise and, in particular, the 50 cycle a.c. noise as well as movement and muscle artefacts. Murray in 1992 validated measurements obtained with this system against direct measurements in the raw signals.

The clinician is faced with the interpretation of an immense amount of information that has to be processed in a continuous form by the use of the concept of a weighted running average (Rhyne, 1968). This allows for continuous updating of the average. All complexes are given a weighting that is highest with the most recent complex. Signal-to-noise ratio serves as a filter against poor quality signals by only accepting a ratio above 3:1. Marvell and Kirk in 1980 described a line-fit routine to enable the location of the waveform components. The up and down slopes of the rising and falling edge of the waveform are calculated by linear regression and the apex of the intersection can be used to assess the position of the peak of the wave (e.g. P or R wave) and the beginning of the wave can be calculated from the point of intersection with the baseline.

The regression line-fit routine is shown in Fig. 4.12. The regression lines form the basis for the calculation of 18 FECG temporal and morphological characteristics. Measurements and calculations are performed every two seconds and stored with the raw FECG. The definitions are listed in Table 4.1 (see Chapter 4). It can be seen that some of the definitions are not those that are used in adult electrocardiography. For example, the PR interval in the fetus is described as the duration of time between the peak of the P wave and the peak of the R wave. This has been shown to bear a strong correlation with the traditional PQ interval but has the particular advantage of being robust and consistent.

The PR Interval and the PR/FHR Relationship

Studies on the P wave are not new and indeed have been investigated extensively since the introduction of scalp electrodes in the 1950s and have been reviewed in the Chapter 1.

Much of the work up to the 1970s was beset with technical difficulties. However, Pardi's animal studies in 1971 were important in quantifying changes in the PQ interval in fetal lambs in relation to graded reductions in oxygen tension, and they showed that the PQ intervals were prolonged in the asphyxiated fetus.

Yeh's work on fetal baboons (1975) was based on cord compression that in itself produces specific haemodynamic changes. These studies showed that the PR interval was prolonged during episodes of bradycardia but neither Pardi nor Yeh looked directly at the correlations with heart rate, and in the light of subsequent studies, the relationship of specific time intervals with heart rate is critical.

P Wave Morphology and Area

Several investigators have demonstrated changes in the morphology characterised by inversion, notching and disappearance. Prolongation of the PQ interval as described by Pardi *et al.* (1974) was found to be associated with mild late decelerations and it was suggested at that time that this prolongation could be the result of mild vagal stimulation leading to suppression of the atrioventricular conduction system.

Mohajer *et al.* (1995) noticed that, using the Nottingham system, P wave area and amplitude appeared to diminish and disappear during episodes of profound bradycardia. Examination of the raw complexes showed that the P wave had not disappeared and was still present but no longer bore any relationship to the R wave, thus indicating a complete disruption of conduction between the SA node and the AV node, and a second- or third-degree heart block which may have a hypoxic basis (see Fig. 1.6). Inversion and notching of the P wave do not appear to bear any relationship to respiratory acidosis and hypoxia in the fetus.

The duration of the P wave and the P wave area were shown to have a relationship with respiratory acidaemia in the fetus (Jenkins, 1984) and also to have a weak correlation with umbilical venous noradrenaline levels (Murray, 1992). However, both the P wave duration and wave area showed weak correlations only with fetal acidaemia at birth and are not of any practical value for clinical use.

The PR/FHR Relationship

In his PhD thesis in 1982, Family applied cross-correlation techniques to a large number of variables of the fetal ECG to see if any previously unknown relationships might emerge in both normal and hypoxaemic fetuses.

Apart from those relationships that were self-evident, the most consistent feature in the normal fetus was an inverse correlation between the PR interval and heart rate. Such a relationship had previously been demonstrated in the adult by Atterhog *et al.* in 1977 where the PR interval was studied in relation to heart rate during exercise.

Murray (1986) then demonstrated that the relationship changes to a positive correlation where there is fetal compromise and hypoxaemia, and the PR interval shortens. Murray (1992) hypothesised that, in the normal fetus, mild hypoxaemia induces an increase in the adrenaline levels which causes an increase in heart rate and shortening of the PR interval. On the other hand, increasing hypoxaemia affects the slow oxygen-dependent channels of the SA node, thereby reducing heart rate, whilst the increasing levels of adrenaline will continue to shorten the PR interval.

In his initial clinical studies in 1986, Murray recorded the FECG using the Nottingham system in 155 women and showed that, whilst changes in the PR/RR correlation from positive to negative were common, a persistently negative relationship was commonly seen to be associated with a fall in cord arterial blood pH from 7.32 in those infants where the PR/RR

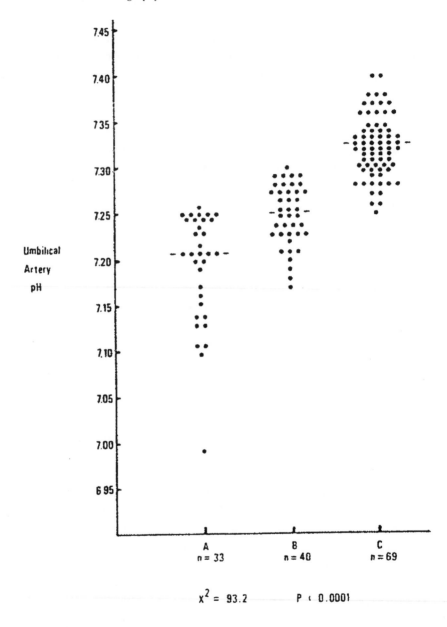

Fig. 6.1. Changes in the FECG complex correlated with cord arterial blood pH. Group C = PR/ RR positive; Group B = PR/RR negative; Group A = PR/RR negative + ST segment elevated (reprinted with permission from Murray, 1986; copyright © Walter de Gruyter GmbH & Co. KG).

relationship remained positive throughout labour down to 7.24 in the negative group. Where this latter group was subdivided by the additional presence of an alteration of the ST segment in relation to the R wave height by more than 5%, the mean cord arterial pH fell to a range of 6.99–7.26. The scatter of the data are illustrated in Fig. 6.1.

It can, however, be seen that there is a considerable scatter of the data and this is a critical issue when seeking to apply these observations to routine clinical practice. These observations were essentially confirmed in both chronically and acutely asphyxiated fetal lambs (Murray, 1992; Widmark *et al.*, 1992).

The PR interval can be altered by other factors, such as local anaesthetic drugs used in epidural analgesia, that have a direct effect on the fetal myocardial conduction system although this does not appear to affect the PR/FHR correlation.

Morgan and Symonds (1991) showed from fetal data collected during labour that the PR interval differs between male and female fetuses. The interval was longer in males at term and the QRS width was also longer. This may be the result of weight differences between male and female infants. The mean heart rate in the male infants was higher than in the females and it has been postulated that the higher rates in the male fetus may be as a result of higher sympathetic tone in males.

Wijngaarden *et al.* (1996) explored the PR/FHR relationship during fetal compromise in chronically instrumented sheep to try and improve our understanding of this relationship. Under strictly controlled circumstances in a study of 20 chronically instrumented fetal lambs, an implanted balloon occluder was placed around the maternal common iliac artery and silver electrodes were implanted into the lambs. Three to five days later, stepwise occlusion of the common iliac artery was performed until fetal hypoxia was induced and fetal oxygen content was reduced to 35% of the previous steady state levels. The fetal ECG was recorded and replayed on a Racal Store 4 tape recorder for subsequent analysis. The cord arterial pH fell to 7.15 indicating a similar level of acidosis found in the human fetus when subjected to fetal hypoxia.

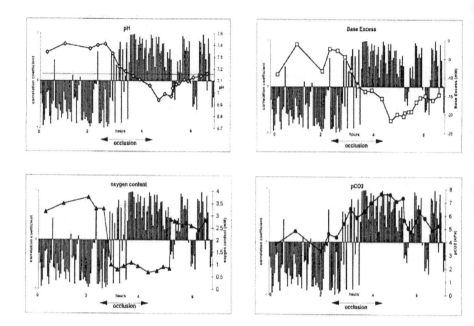

Fig. 6.2. Response to induced fetal hypoxaemia in the fetal lamb showing the correlation co-efficient changes for PR/FHR following occlusion of the maternal common illiac artery (reprinted with permission from Van Wijngaarden *et al.*, 1996; copyright © Mosby, Inc.).

In the final analysis, four of the 20 animals were excluded for various technical reasons. The differences between the linear correlation values (*r* values) were noted. Fourteen of the 16 sheep studied showed conversion from a negative *r* value to a positive *r* value, thus far, with increasing acidaemia. A typical example of the recorded changes biochemically and biophysically is shown in Fig. 6.2.

The changes in the conduction index are seen in relation to pH, base excess, oxygen content and pCO_2. The authors point out that mature fetal lambs premedicated with atropine still respond to hypoxaemia by reversal of the normally negative PR/FHR relationship and thus a vagal cause for this relationship seems unlikely. The authors suggest that the changing PR/FHR relationship during fetal compromise is due to the different responses of the SA node and the AV node to hypoxaemia. The authors also suggest that depolarisation of the SA node results from the declining membrane potential of the pacemaker cells reaching a trigger level at which time there is a dramatic increase in Na^+ ion influx and K^+ ion efflux. At the same time, an increase in membrane permeability results in an influx of Ca^{++} ions. They noted that the time between the start of occlusion and the onset of fetal acidosis varied considerably.

In 1998, Westgate *et al.* published a further study using a sheep model but, on this occasion, they used cord occlusion rather than occlusion of the uterine artery and showed that the initial switch from positive to negative (PR/RR) following cord occlusion was demonstrated. However, this was followed by a return to positive even in the presence of severe acidosis and would appear to be at variance from those reported in Van Wijngaarden's work. One possible explanation could be the differences in vascular haemodynamic changes occurring during cord compression versus that of common iliac compression. Nevertheless, the change in the PR/RR relationship reported by Westgate *et al.* confirmed the observations previously reported by Murray and others. Westgate *et al.* also noted in their experimental model that the change in the relationship was relatively consistent for the first 30 minutes from the onset of the occlusions but subsequently became unstable. The duration of the change in the PR/RR relationship and the fact that the relationship subsequently reverted back could probably be explained by differences in occlusion and recovery periods used, thereby allowing the fetus to recompensate after each short-term acute hypoxic insult. If one extrapolates from the explanation postulated by Westgate, then it could be assumed that every deceleration would produce a change in the PR/RR relationship, limiting its clinical usefulness.

In applying all these observations to the monitoring of the human fetus, there is a need to develop systems that do not over-interpret data and reproduce the failures that have arisen in cardiotocography where the system has high sensitivity but low specificity.

Murray (1992) introduced the term "conduction index". This is a continually updated expression of Pearson's correlation coefficient of the PR interval and the filtered FHR. If it is positive for more than 20 minutes, then it has been found to be related to fetal deterioration. To stabilise these measurements on a longer-term basis, Mohajer *et al.* (1994) introduced the term "ratio index" which is calculated by multiplying the normalised PR interval of the total recording time by the time that this product has exceeded two positive standard deviations of its own mean. This calculation, which is expressed as a percentage of "abnormality time" within the total time, is likely to reflect chronic fetal deterioration in contrast to the conduction index which reflects more acute changes.

The Application of PR/FHR to Clinical Trials

The initial studies on the role of the PR/FHR correlation as termed the conduction index were necessarily descriptive. Murray (1986), in the first studies on the use of this system, found that when the conduction index was positive for longer than 20 minutes, there was a significant risk of acute fetal compromise in the form of abnormal umbilical artery blood gas measurements. However, this was also reinforced by the assessment of a shift in the ST segment that enhanced the accuracy of prediction.

However, Mohajer and others in 1994 suggested further novel approaches to attempt to quantify with greater precision the amount of total time in any given labour that the relationship strayed outside the normal range.

This was a retrospective study and the term "ratio index" was introduced. The procedure depends on establishing an initial normal baseline for FHR and PR, but once this is established, the ratio index is expressed as a percentage of total recording time and is defined as the times that $Z^{FHR} \times Z^{PR}$ exceed two standard deviations of the average expressed as a percentage of the total recording time in which Z^{FHR} and Z^{PR} are the standardised values for FHR and PR time-interval measurements.

The Z-transformed product for both FHR and PR was calculated as follows:

$$Z^{FHR} = \frac{(FHR - FHR\ mean)}{FHR^{sd}},$$

where Z^{FHR} is the Z-transformed value for the fetal heart rate at time 1; FHR mean is the mean value of the FHR over the whole labour; and FHR^{sd}

is the standard deviation of the FHR over the whole labour.

A similar calculation is made for the PR interval so that the Z transform is:

$$Z^{PR} = \frac{(PR - PR \, mean)}{PR^{sd}}.$$

The relationship between the ratio index and umbilical artery pH was significant ($r = -0.38$, $p < 0.01$) as was the relationship with lactate ($r = 0.36$, $p < 0.01$), $\log_{10}$ norepinephrine ($r = 0.37$, $p < 0.01$) and hypoxanthine ($r = 0.28$, $p < 0.01$). The authors concluded that the ratio index might be useful in clinical practice and that a ratio index in excess of 4% was associated with the development of fetal acidosis.

In 1996, Reed *et al.* reported a retrospective study on 250 high-risk labours to try and identify whether the use of standard EFM (cardiotocography) combined with the FECG parameters would have superior predictive capacity as compared to standard EFM by itself. The EFM plus FECG arm was based on FHR, conduction index (CI) and ratio index (RI). A positive CI for longer than 20 minutes and a RI greater than 4% were defined as abnormal and if two of the three indicators were considered abnormal, then fetal blood sampling or expedited delivery were indicated. This was a large study and showed that the combined assessment reduced the number of fetal blood samples being carried out from 85.6–26.8% with a simultaneous reduction in unsuspected acidaemia at the time of the delivery. However, these studies were retrospective and, whilst promising, it was clear that further randomised prospective studies should be performed to ascertain whether the use of the FECG parameters would reduce intervention rates while maintaining enhanced safety in terms of prediction of fetal condition at birth.

Prospective Trials

In an effort to ratify these earlier findings, Wijngaarden and his colleagues (1996) established a randomised prospective study on 214 women with high-risk pregnancies. The patients were divided into two groups. One group was monitored by EFM alone whilst the other group was monitored by EFM plus fetal ECG analysis. As with the previous studies of Reed and Mohajer, the Nottingham fetal ECG analyser was used. Decisions were made solely by the on-call labour ward staff. Intervention with the EFM group was based on the guidelines laid down by the International Federation of Obstetrics and Gynecology. Intervention consisted of fetal blood sampling or delivery. The group monitored by FHR plus the fetal ECG was assessed on the basis of the CTG, conduction index and ratio index. If two of the three criteria were judged to be abnormal, i.e. conduction index positive for more than 20 minutes, ratio index greater than 4% and FHR abnormal, then a fetal blood sampling or delivery was indicated. There was an "opt-out" clause for prolonged and profound bradycardia. Outcome measures were based firstly on interventions such as the number and results of fetal blood samples and the number and types of operative interventions and their indications. Fetal condition was based on arterial and venous cord blood acid–base parameters, Apgar scores at 1, 5 and 10 minutes, and neonatal resuscitation plus pathology in the first month of life as well as admissions to neonatal intensive care units. The umbilical cord arterial blood was classified as acidotic at delivery if the pH was < 7.15. A total of 214 subjects were included in the trial but 30 were excluded because of an inability to obtain an analysable signal, non-availability of cord blood measurements and discontinuity of the trial. The management instructions are shown in Table 6.1.

Table 6.1. Management criteria for the randomised study on EFM versus EFM + FECG (reprinted with permission from Van Wijngaarden et al., 1996; copyright © Mosby, Inc.).

	EFM normal		EFM abnormal	
FECG criteria	RI < 4% and CI pos < 20 min	RI > = 4% and Ci pos > = 20 min	RI < 4% and CI pos < 20 min	RI > = 4% or CI pos > = 20 min
Action	None	FBS or delivery	None	FBS or delivery

The results showed that 28 patients in the EFM group alone had FBS samples taken as compared with only five in the EFM/FECG group — a difference that was statistically significant. According to the cord blood samples, significant acidosis was missed in nine cases as compared with four in the FECG group. In the EFM group, 27 of the 28 scalp samples taken were normal whereas in the FECG group, only three of the five were normal.

The number of assisted deliveries was similar in both groups, although in the EFM group, the number of assisted deliveries for presumed fetal distress was 16/42 as compared with 7 of 36 in the FECG group. The authors concluded that the addition of FECG analysis to conventional EFM significantly reduced the need for scalp blood sampling without increasing the risk to the fetus. There was still clearly a need for a much bigger study.

Strachan *et al.* (2000) have published a further retrospective analysis of the FECG in 679 cases in women recruited as part of a prospective randomised trial and as part of observational studies with evaluation of the FECG during the last 30 minutes preceding delivery. This study included an analysis of the PR/FHR ratio and the T/QRS ratio and, using receiver operator curves, calculated the sensitivity, specificity, positive predictive value, negative predictive value and chi-square for this value. Using a cord arterial pH < = 7.15 and a base excess < = −8 mmol/l as evidence of significant acidaemia, the authors showed that a significant relationship existed between measurements made using the time interval analysis (PR/FHR) but that no such relationship could be demonstrated using the morphology of the FECG (ST segment and T wave height).

However, in a large multicentre randomised trial of cardiotocography alone versus cardiotocography plus PR interval analysis of the fetal ECG in which 1038 high-risk labours were studied, the same authors could only show a trend towards a reduction in operative intervention in the FECG group and no difference in the incidence of unsuspected acidaemia. When Wijngaarden and his colleagues subsequently reanalysed these data, they showed that protocol was of such a standard in this trial that cases randomised to both arms of the trial appeared to have been managed by conventional electronic fetal monitoring which in a sense largely invalidated the trial.

The QRS Complex

Essentially, there are two measurements that can be utilised and these are:

(i) the width and shape of the QRS complex;
(ii) the vectors as assessed by the R/S relationship.

The width of the QRS complex is probably the most robust of all ECG measurements but also the least revealing. Most changes in morphology are either agonal or not significant and so they have not proven to be particularly useful clinically. The QRS duration represents the time for the action potential to spread through the ventricles. It is a short time that provides a highly stable and reproducible event.

The relationship with gestational age is highly significant as is the relationship with birth weight (Morgan and Symonds, 1991), and the QRS time is longer in males than in females. Brambati and Pardi showed in 1980 that QRS duration is related to myocardial mass. The mass of the male heart as with body weight is larger than in the female and, therefore, the QRS complex is wider. Morgan and Symonds (1991) also showed that the QRS width was unaffected by uterine activity. Lee and Blackwell in 1974 suggested that shortening of the QRS duration occurred in relation to early and late decelerations but no other workers have confirmed these observations and no correlation has been found between fetal compromise and QRS duration.

The R/S Ratio and Fetal Vector Cardiography

The early work of Larks and Larks (1965) was based on observations made from signals obtained from the maternal abdomen and, therefore, any verification of the theoretical axis measurements could not be validated against direct fetal or neonatal measurements. Yet this work had a reasonable theoretical basis and was essentially confirmed in terms of vector analysis in the neonate and with subsequent observations made by Symonds.

In 1972, he showed an association of cardiac axis shift to the left in the presence of fetal acidosis and hyperkalaemia and this appeared to have the potential as a clinical tool. However, any value that would accrue from these observations would have to be achieved within any particular labour in the knowledge that moving the placement of the scalp electrode might change the shape of the waveform and, therefore, it would be most effective in the context of a constant electrode position and by assessing changes that occurred in labour on a temporal basis. The theory behind this method of approach is rather unattractive because it is only possible to use a two-dimensional electrode system to measure a three-dimensional phenomenon. Carretti *et al.* (1989) reported four cases in which increased QRS complex voltages or deviation of the mean electrical axis occurred following the administration of large doses of oxytocin where the electrical axis shifted to the left. However, in view of the hyperstimulation of uterine activity, it is difficult to equate these changes only with hypoxia as there would be substantial changes in the pattern of vascular pressures in the fetus.

Nevertheless, it is surprising that the topic has not been pursued with more vigour.

The QT Interval and the ST Segment

In the light of changes that occur in T wave configuration in adult myocardial ischaemia, it is not surprising that this has been considered a high priority area in fetal research. It is often difficult to measure precisely the point of intersection of the T wave with the baseline. Nevertheless, in a study using visual assessment, Symonds in 1971 showed that the QT interval correlated strongly and positively with R–R′ duration and there was a prolongation in the presence of fetal acidosis.

Lee and Blackwell (1974) reported that the QT interval shortened in some cases of fetal acidosis and, in animal studies using fetal lambs, Pardi (1971) demonstrated that hypoxia in the lamb was associated with elevation of the ST segment. Rosen and Kjellmer in 1975 showed, with experiments in guinea pigs, that ST waveform changes and a progressive increase of the T wave height occurred with induced hypoxia before the onset of bradycardia. Hokegard *et al.* in 1981 reported work on metabolic studies in fetal lambs with surface biopsies from the epicardial surface and demonstrated that glycogen, creatinine phosphate, ATP and lactate levels changed during hypoxia and a decrease in high energy substrates was associated with increases in T wave amplitude. This work formed the basis for much of the subsequent work on the T/QRS ratio. Jenkins *et al.* (1986), in a study involving a cohort of 14 normal fetuses and 10 with significant fetal acidosis at delivery,showed that a long-term increase in the ST segment and T wave height was associated with fetal acidosis.

The T/QRS Ratio

Measurements based on the morphology of the waveform present particular difficulties because of the use of single electrode systems. Nevertheless, as previously reviewed in Chapter 1, extensive clinical trials have now been performed on the basis of morphologic changes in configuration of the T wave and the ST segment as expressed by the T/QRS ratio.

The clinical work was based on a considerable volume of work produced in animal experiments. In 1982, Greene and others reported work in fetal lambs where they studied the ST waveform in ten chronically instrumented fetal lambs at 115 days to term and described the amplitude of the T wave relative to the amplitude of the QRS complex, thus describing the T/QRS ratio. The T/QRS value was normally less than 0.3. Hypoxia was induced for 1–2.5 hours by administering 7–9% oxygen and 3% CO_2 in nitrogen. Both fetal and maternal blood samples were taken to analyse acid–base and lactate values. The studies showed that when hypoxaemia was induced, the mean T/QRS rose from 0.17–0.59 and reverted to normal when the hypoxaemia was reversed. There was also a strong correlation of the T/QRS ratio to the rate of rise of lactate. An example of the experimental data is shown in Fig. 6.3.

Further studies by Widmark *et al.* in 1988 on fetal lambs, but using a model where hypoxia was induced by compression of the maternal aorta, demonstrated a linear correlation between the T/QRS ratio and plasma epinephrine levels in the mature fetal lamb. Again, the increase in the T wave amplitude was seen with increasing hypoxaemia.

The largest clinical trial so far performed in this field is the Plymouth trial

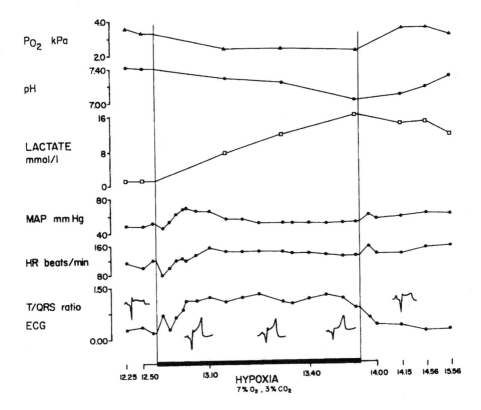

Fig. 6.3. Changes in the T/QRS ratio during a one hour experiment on a fetal lamb. The increase in the T/QRS ratio is clearly apparent although this ratio is different from that seen in the human fetus (reprinted with permission from Greene *et al.*, 1982; copyright © Mosby, Inc.).

in 1993 which was a study of 2400 high-risk pregnancies where patients were randomised to standard CTG monitoring or to CTG plus the T/QRS ratio. A T/QRS ratio was considered to be normal if the value fell between 0.05–0.24. Values between 0.24–0.5 were considered to be of intermediate grade and values in excess of 0.5 were considered to be abnormal. These values were considered in conjunction with the CTG and a fixed protocol recommended either no action, fetal blood sampling or delivery. The total number of deliveries for fetal distress in the CTG group was 111 and the figure for the CTG + T/QRS group was six, a difference that was highly significant ($p < 0.001$). This reduction was not achieved at the expense of a significant increase in the number of infants with birth asphyxia although it should be noted that the number of infants born with cord artery pH values of < 7.15 was 110 in the CTG + T/QRS group as compared with 101 in the CTG only group. However, there was no difference in the numbers with severe acidosis using a cut-off point of pH < 7.05.

Some anxieties about the validity of the recording systems have been raised by the study of Skillern (1994) when a comparative study of the two ECG analysis systems currently in use (the Stan system from Gothenburg and the FECG analyser from Nottingham) was reported using signals generated by a computer and those obtained and recorded from ten fetuses during labour. There was satisfactory concordance where the signal was generated by a computer but the analysis of biologically obtained signals showed poor concordance and it was considered that the difference in T/QRS values was probably due to differences in reference points for the measurement of the ST segment and T wave height.

Since this study, the original Stan system from Sweden has been modified and new digital filters have been introduced, which significantly reduce baseline wander without destroying the ST information. Further multicentre trials are now underway.

In 1995, de Haan *et al.* undertook further sheep studies using the Stan system. They examined the ST waveform and the T/QRS ratio in response to asphyxia induced by gradual and graded reductions in uterine blood flow in sheep where the gestational age fell between 113–132 days. Fetal arterial oxygen saturation was reduced to 35% of the baseline values and this was sustained for one hour, during which time the fetal blood pH fell. Twenty-two animals survived more than 12 hours of asphyxia. Animals were also pretreated with an adenosine transport inhibitor or a calcium channel blocker to try and minimise the effects of the asphyxia but these drugs did not affect survival. The maximum T/QRS ratios were reached at the peak of asphyxia. However, the sensitivity and specificity for predicting hypoxaemia or acidaemia were 24% and 42.6%, and 25.1% and 45.3%, respectively. The authors concluded that in fetal lambs, the T/QRS ratio failed to predict fetal hypoxaemia and fetal acidosis.

This work was strongly attacked by Rosen and Westgate (1996) who pointed out that signal quality had not been assessed and the electrode placements were not the same as those used in previous experimental work. They also claimed that many of the animals exhibited chronically elevated waveforms before the onset of hypoxia and the application of linear regression to the analysis was inappropriate. De Haan replied by pointing out that the Stan recorder checks its own quality and that the objective of the study was to ascertain the diagnostic power of the T/QRS ratio to predict fetal well-being and in particular to look at the assessment during periods of stable heart rate rather than during episodes of bradycardia.

The issue of the value of the current use of the FECG morphological characteristics and time intervals for the prediction of fetal compromise remains promising but unresolved.

Chapter 7

FETAL CARDIAC ARRHYTHMIAS

Disorders of Cardiac Rhythms in the Fetus

In the normal heart, depolarisation follows activation of the sino-atrial node. When depolarisation originates in other parts of the myocardium or the conduction system is blocked at some point, then disorders of rhythm occur. The same principles are obtained in the fetal heart with the difference that the mother controls the fetal environment, and that the frequency of occurrence of different abnormalities follows a different profile in the fetus.

Cardiac arrhythmias have their origins in three places:

— the atrial muscle;
— the region around the AV node, i.e. nodal or junctional;
— the ventricular muscle.

Sinus rhythm, atrial rhythm and junctional or nodal rhythm are classified as supraventricular rhythms. The depolarisation wave spreads to the ventricles in the normal way and, therefore, the QRS complex is normal and narrow with the exceptions of bundle branch block and complete heart block that are associated with ventricular escape. Ventricular rhythms, on the other hand, are the result of depolarisation waves initiated in the ventricle wall with a slower pathway through the conduction system, and the QRS complex is wide and abnormal.

The types of abnormal rhythms are classified as:

— the escape rhythms,
— extrasystoles;

— the tachycardias;
— fibrillation.

By far, the commonest abnormalities seen in the fetus are the extrasystoles.

Extrasystoles

This chapter is based on observations made by fetal electrocardiography and not on the detection of arrhythmias by ultrasonography where the literature is extensive.

Extrasystoles can arise from the initiation of depolarisation in any part of the heart. The extrasystoles or "éctopic" beats may be atrial or nodal extrasystoles in which case they are known as *supraventricular extrasystoles* or they may arise within the ventricle, in which case, they are known as *ventricular extrasystoles*.

Supraventricular Extrasystoles

By far, the commonest abnormalities reported in the literature in fetal cardiac arrhythmias are the extrasystoles. There have been a large number of individual case reports and several substantial reports reviewing large series of cases. Where there are multiple extrasystoles, they interfere with effective

Table 7.1. Reported extrasystoles

Author	Year	Cases	Supraventricular	Ventricular	Outcome
Hon and Huang	1962	25	23	2	All normal[+]
Komaromy *et al.*	1977	47	38	9	All normal[*]
Sugarman *et al.*	1978	7	6	1	All normal
Young *et al.*	1979	15	13	2	All normal
Maragnes *et al.*	1991	69	N.A.	N.A.	All normal

[+]all normal within 48 hours
[*]except one case with cord venous pH of 7.17

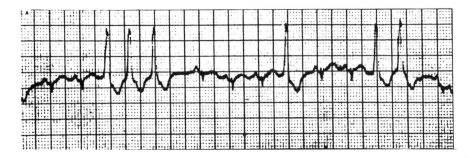

Fig. 7.1. Direct FECG recording showing ventricular extrasystoles with atrial trigeminy (reprinted with permission from Young *et al.*, 1979; copyright © American College of Obstetricians and Gynecologists).

fetal monitoring as all systems that record heart rate in standard cardiotocography are unable to cope with grossly irregular short-term variations in heart rate. An analysis of some of the major series is shown in Table 7.1. It is apparent from all these studies that extrasystoles in the fetus do not carry any sinister significance. An example of ventricular extrasystoles associated with atrial trigeminy is shown in Fig. 7.1.

Management

It follows from these observations that it is not necessary or appropriate to intervene where extrasystoles occur, whether they are supraventricular or ventricular. However, when there is an obvious cause for the extrasystoles, then that cause should be removed. Oei, Vosters and van der Hagen (1989) reported three cases of excessive maternal caffeine intake. In the first case, the fetus exhibited frequent blocked extrasystoles resulting in bradycardia. The mother had drunk ten cups of coffee during the hours before delivery and the babies urine was shown to contain caffeine. The extrasystoles stopped spontaneously after three days. In the second case, a woman was admitted at term with a history that she had drunk 1.5 litres of cola daily for the two weeks prior to admission and, on admission, the fetal heart beat was irregular although it was known to have been normal three weeks prior to admission. The ECG showed the presence of multiple extrasystoles.

Within three days after delivery, the heartbeat was normal.

In the third case, the mother was admitted to hospital at 23 weeks because the fetus was noted to have a totally irregular heart beat. The mother stated that she drank 1.5 litres of cola per day together with two cups of coffee and one cup of cocoa. She was advised to stop and, within one week, the arrhythmia had disappeared.

It would seem sensible therefore to advise mothers under these circumstances to avoid high caffeine intakes. The only other difficulty that may arise in labour is that it may not be possible to monitor the fetal heart rate and, therefore, the condition of the fetus must be monitored by the use of scalp blood sampling.

Escape Rhythms — The Bradycardias

Bradycardia in the fetus is defined as a heart rate of less than 110 beats/minute and may be classified as:

— sinus bradycardia;
— blocked atrial premature beats;
— complete heart block.

Sinus Bradycardia

Although most episodes are of short duration and are associated with cord compression and commonly seen during labour, there is a small group of fetuses that exhibit a persistently slow heart rate with a 1:1 atrioventricular concordance which may be identified either antenatally or during the course of labour. Where the heartbeat exhibits both bradycardia and irregularity, it is likely that there are blocked atrial premature beats.

Management

Short-term episodes of bradycardia are a common feature of labour and are discussed in the context of the management of fetal hypoxia. The presence of a persistent bradycardia that is due to a low setting of the heart rate is an uncommon event, but provided that there is evidence of some heart rate variability and there is ultrasound evidence of normal fetal activity, there are no grounds for intervention and conservative management is indicated. These abnormalities in rate are generally identified antenatally.

Blocked Atrial Premature Beats

This condition is usually benign and does not need treatment. The premature beats usually disappear within four days after delivery and are not associated with any cardiac anomalies.

Complete Heart Block

Unlike the previous arrhythmias described, complete heart block has serious implications for the fetus. In a recent review by Copel and Kleinman (1997), the authors pointed out that approximately 50% of all fetuses with complete heart block have major structural anomalies that tend to involve the atrioventricular junction. The remaining fetuses with complete heart block are mainly associated with the presence of abnormal auto-antibodies in the maternal circulation.

The association between systemic lupus erythematosis and heart block was noted as long ago as 1962 by Larks and Anderson when they recorded an abnormally widened QRS complex from a maternal abdominal ECG and speculated at that time that the abnormal complex might be associated with "some internal environmental factors for this fetus". Gross *et al.* (1989) examined the relationship between maternal connective tissue diseases with specific auto-antibodies and showed that there was a high association between the presence of anti-La and anti-Ro and the presence of complete congenital heart block. These antibodies appear to have a particular affinity for the fetal conduction system and this interaction leads to an inflammatory response. Immune heart block may lead to cardiac failure and the development of non-immune hydrops.

Management

Copel, Buyon and Kleinman (1994) have reported the treatment of five cases of complete heart block by the administration of dexamethasone to the mother in a dose of 4 mg orally daily with the resolution of non-immune hydrops in two fetuses and the reversion of a second-degree to a first degree block in a third infant. These lesions do not appear before 24 weeks gestation.

Alternative methods of treatment include the administration of amiodarone and flecainide to the mother but this may expose the mother to the pro-arrhythmic effects of these drugs and, therefore, it is advisable to adopt extreme caution before giving these drugs. Some attempts have been made to use transvenous pacing but so far without success.

The Tachycardias

Fetal tachycardia is generally defined as a rate in excess of 160 beats per minute. However, for purposes of the definition of arrhythmias, it is better to use a figure of 180 beats per minute. The tachycardias may be supra-ventricular or ventricular in origin.

Supraventricular Tachycardias

The AV node cannot conduct atrial discharges in rates in excess of 200 beats per minute and, above this rate, the AV node protects the ventricles from very fast activation and hence inefficient action.

Supraventricular tachycardia (SVT) is the most common form of this type of tacchyarrythmia and are commonly of a re-entrant type. An extrasystole leads to a circular movement of electrical impulses from the region of the AV junction re-entering the atrium via an accessory conduction pathway. The fetus will have a normal electrocardiogram during most cases because the accessory pathway does not conduct impulses in an antegrade direction. If there is antegrade conduction through the accessory pathway, then the ECG will exhibit a short PR interval, a delta wave and a broadened

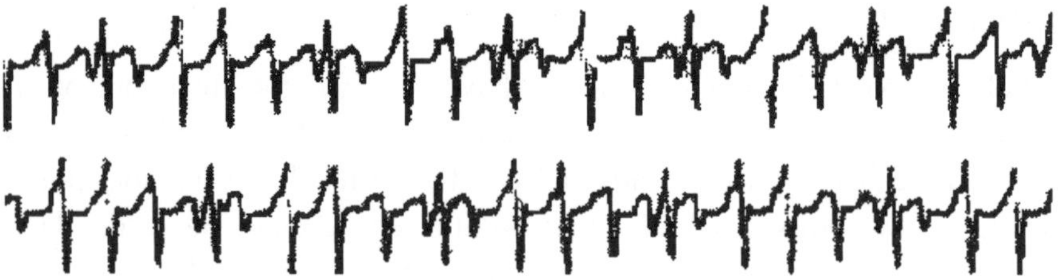

Fig. 7.2. FECG obtained by scalp electrode in the late first stage of labour. The ECG showed evidence of a nodal tachycardia with a wandering pacemaker (reprinted with permission from Symonds, 1972; copyright © ANZJOG).

QRS complex. These are the findings seen in the Wolff–Parkinson–White syndrome. The changes become apparent after conversion. These abnormalities may be episodic but they may be persistent and associated with hydrops. The heart rate is usually between 240–260 beats per minute.

Symonds in 1972 described a case of nodal tachycardia with a heart rate of 190 beats/minute and evidence from the FECG of a wandering pacemaker (Fig. 7.2). At delivery, the cord arterial blood showed a pH of 7.16 and a base excess of −10 mEq/l.

The infant was depressed at birth with an Apgar score of 2 at one minute and showed signs of cardiac failure with an enlarged liver and spleen. The child was digitalised and steadily improved over the following week. By the end of the first year of life, the child was normal and there seems little doubt that the initial arrhythmia was due to fetal acidosis. There was no evidence of any maternal disease.

Management

Copel and Kleinman (1997) have emphasised the importance of assessing the amount of time spent in tachycardia, and the presence or absence of signs of heart failure in the form of hydrops. Short periods of arrhythmia in the absence of hydrops do not need to be treated but prolonged SVT may lead to cardiac failure and death. These authors concluded that treatment with digoxin should be the first line of treatment in the pre-term hydropic fetus.

They recommend a maternal loading dose, given intravenously, of 0.5 mg to be followed by two 0.25 mg doses at six hourly intervals. Both the mother and fetus are monitored continuously. A total dose of up to 2.0 mg may be required over 36 hours and maternal serum digoxin levels of 1.5 – 2.0 ng/ml are considered ideal, provided no maternal toxicity occurs. Direct treatment by either intramuscular or IV administration has been recorded by Weiner and Thompson (1988), but this has not become the primary approach to treatment. The second line of treatment is with flecainide but this should be used with great caution because of the potential pro-arrhythmic effects.

Atrial Flutter and Atrial Fibrillation

Atrial flutter is a rare complication and has been documented in the literature since the early 1970s. Symonds (1972), shown in Fig. 7.3, recorded a single case of atrial flutter occurring during late labour in an otherwise uneventful pregnancy.

The fetal ECG showed evidence of atrial flutter with a 2:1, 3:1 block. The fetus was mildly acidotic at birth with a cord arterial pH at birth of 7.11 but a neonatal ECG performed four hours after birth was completely normal.

Copel and Kleinman (1997) reported a series of 17 cases, five of which had congenital heart disease and nine exhibited hydrops fetalis. Four of

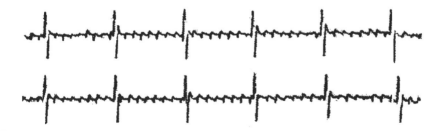

Fig. 7.3. Fetal ECG recorded in late first stage showing changes consistent with atrial flutter (reprinted with permission from Symonds, 1972; copyright © ANZJOG).

these infants died so the condition, although rare, seems to have sinister connotations. Atrial fibrillation is even rarer than flutter and does not appear to be associated with congestive heart failure (Pinsky *et al.*, 1991).

Management

As with SVT, the management is with digoxin but the prognosis is poor in the presence of hydrops. Digoxin should slow conduction at the AV node. It may then be necessary to add in agents such as procainamide or flecainide.

Ventricular Tachycardia

This is a very rare arrhythmia. Ventricular tachycardia arises from a focus of depolarisation with high frequency in the ventricle. It is characterised by rapid but wide QRS complexes. There may be a 1:1 atrioventricular relationship because of retrograde atrial activation. If the fetus is not hydropic and the heart looks structurally normal, then the condition should not be treated.

In premature fetuses, the use of digoxin should be avoided and it may be appropriate to treat the condition with direct umbilical infusion of lidocaine or procainamide followed by maternal therapy with procainamide or propanolol. This therapy should only be used if there is evidence of congestive cardiac failure.

Chapter 8

INFORMATION INTERPRETATION AND TRANSFORMATION

Fetal ECG signals consist of a continuing stream of voltage measurements, so a lot of computing is necessary before they can be used. In addition to the conversion from voltage measurements into the ECG waveform, the computer can be used to enhance the interpretation and clinical use of the data. The functions of the computer in this regard can broadly be divided into three related areas: the transformation of data, the organisation of information and the presentation of the result.

The Transformation of Data

Simple transformations

Transformation converts data from one domain to another and is made to produce information in a more usable form. A primary example is the conversion of a stream of voltage measurement into an ECG waveform, and the conversion of parts of the ECG waveform into the P–R interval and T wave height. The functions used during transformation can be logical or mathematical, and they vary in complexity. These functions may reflect a defined theoretical assumption, or they can be derived empirically modelling a reference set of data.

Transformations based on theoretical assumptions

Algorithms for transformation may be produced, reflecting a theoretical construct that is understood and invariable, such as the logarithmic function $y = \log(x)$. As most biological measurements have an exponential distribution (where the variance increases with the measurements), a logarithmic transformation results in a linear and normally distributed measurement that is easier to use. An example of this is the use of the pH rather than hydrogen ion concentration to measure the level of acidity, as demonstrated in Fig. 8.1.

Another example is using the inverse of the RR interval as heart rate, resulting in a normally distributed linear measurement that is familiar to clinicians.

The Z transform $(Z = (\text{value-mean})/\text{standard deviation})$ converts a measurement into a standard deviation unit. This standardised measurement is useful as widely diverse measurements can be changed into a population-based parameter with similar scalar units, so that statistical comparisons and mathematical integration can be more easily made.

A clinically useful transformation is the logistic transformation $[y = 1/1 - \exp(-x)]$. This converts a measurement into a value between 0 and 1

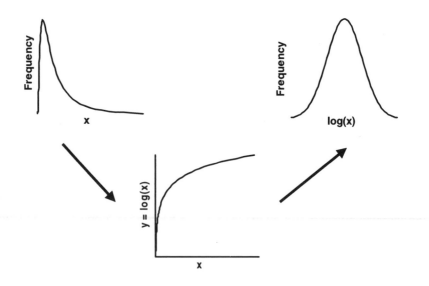

Fig. 8.1. Transformation of the measurement of hydrogen ion concentration to that of acidity.

that can represent either probability or the extent that some decision can be held to be true. This is particularly useful when there is a need to dichotomise a continuous measurement along an arbitrary point, such as creating a measurement for tachycardia from FHR in beats per minute shown in Fig. 8.2. From this, what appears to be a normally distributed heart rate can be transformed into subpopulations of normal and tachycardic heart rates, as shown in Fig. 8.3.

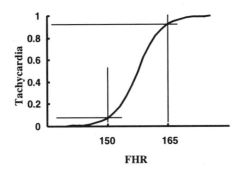

Fig. 8.2. Dichotomisation of heart rate using logistic transformation into a measurement of tachycardia using two fixed points.

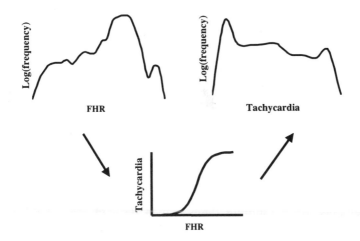

Fig. 8.3. Transformation of a normally distributed heart rate into subpopulations of normal and tachycardic heart rates.

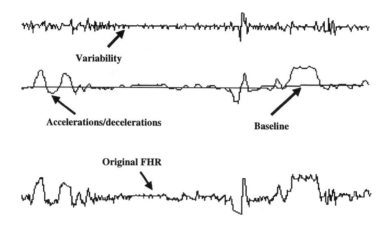

Fig. 8.4. Extraction of heart rate baseline, variability and accelerations by separating the segment of heart rate tracing into defined frequency bands.

Serial transformations

Transformation may be used to convert a series of measurements into a composite measurement. An example is the calculation of the mean and standard deviation of an array of numbers. The creation of a trend measurement from a large number of irregular measurements over a period of time is often used in the analysis of the ECG. An additional useful approach is using frequency analysis techniques such as the fast Fourier transformation (FFT) to decompose a complex waveform into its frequency components.

The CTG is a common example of serial transformation, where a large number of FHR measurements are converted by a complex set of algorithms into baseline, variability, accelerations and decelerations, as demonstrated in Fig. 8.4.

Multivariate transformations

Composite measurements can be produced from a cluster of different measurements, by combining them with a defined algorithm and giving appropriate weighting to each of the measurements. The formulae and weightings used can be derived according to theoretical constructs, or more commonly, they are derived empirically according to the underlying patterns in a reference set of data.

The T/QRS ratios, and the correlation between the PR interval and RR intervals, are two examples of multivariate transformation based on an understanding of the electrophysiology of the fetal heart.

There are two common statistical approaches to define underlying patterns from a reference set of data, from which multivariate transformation can be derived. The first is to analyse the relationship between predictor and outcome measurements, so that future data can fit into these assumed relationships. The second is taxonomy, to identify heterogeneous subgroups within the data set, so that future data can be allocated into the appropriate subgroups.

In data sets where predictor and outcome variables are both present, statistical calculations can be used to produce a formula that best fit the relationship between them. Examples of these are multiple regression analysis, discriminant analysis and Baysean probability analysis. Both multiple regression and Baysean probability analyses have been successfully used to produce a fetal risk index using measurements from the fetal CTG. An example is to measure the area of deceleration that has occurred after a contraction ends and transform that into a risk index, as shown in Fig. 8.5.

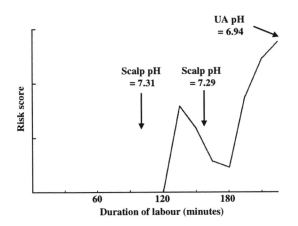

Fig. 8.5. Example of a risk score index that could be produced by combining components of heart rate interpretation, such as baseline, number of decelerations and period of tachycardia. The individual components could, for example, be statistically combined (from Strachan *et al.*, unpublished data).

When there is no outcome measurement in the reference data set, members of the set can be rearranged into clusters so that similarities between members in the same cluster are high while that between clusters are low. This allows different groups that exist in the reference data set to be identified and isolated. An example of this is cluster analysis.

Although these statistical methods are powerful, they are constrained by the assumptions underlying their methodologies. The reference set is assumed to be representative of the population. Measurements are assumed to be linear and normally distributed, and relationships between measurements are assumed to be regular throughout the whole range of each of the measurements. Correlation between any two measurements is also assumed to be independent of any other measurement in the set. Because these assumptions are not always correct, models derived from these calculations often cannot be successfully generalised.

Neural Networks

Neural networks can be used in the place of multivariate statistical methods, both in exploring data and in the construction of composite measurements.

Neural networks belong to a class of problem-solving techniques that simulate the functions of the nervous system. The basic processing unit is a neurone, which processes one or more input signals according to an adaptive algorithm to produce an output signal as demonstrated in Fig. 8.6.

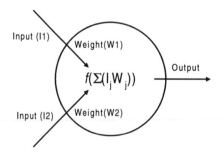

Fig. 8.6. Schematic mathematical representation of a neurone, the basic processing element in a neural network. Inputs (|1, |2) are weighted according to the values of the weights (W1, W2) and then combined mathematically to produce an output.

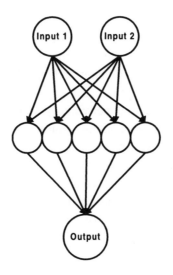

Fig. 8.7. Combination of individual neuronal processing units into a layered structure of inputs, middle processing layers and output.

The neurones are arranged in a network (Fig. 8.7) so that the output from some neurones becomes the input of others, allowing a complex interaction between these neurones and signals. The network can be trained by a reference data set so that the processing algorithm can adapt to produce the desired output. How a trained neural network functions therefore depends on how the reference data set is obtained, how the processing algorithm are made to adapt to the data, and how the neurones are linked together architecturally. Potentially, therefore, an infinite variety of problem-solving methods can be produced.

Although many neural networks have been used in medicine, the two most common types are the back-propagation network (BPN), and the self-organising map (SOM) such as that described by Kohonen in 1984.

The BPN consists of a layer of neurones to receive input signals, a layer to produce output results and one or more middle layers to process data. Input signals to each neurone are weighted, summed and converted by a function into an output value. Outputs from one layer of neurone become the inputs of the next layer, until the output layer is reached. The output results are compared with idealised results in the reference data set to produce corrections for input weightings, and the processes are repeated until the outputs of the network are sufficiently close to that in the reference data set.

The BPN is therefore able to adapt or learn the patterns of relationship between the input and output values in a large data set. Given a sufficiently large network and training, the network is able to adapt to any pattern provided the dataset does not contain contradictory patterns. The method of adaptation is by iterative approximation and is not dependent on any assumption about the nature of the data.

In analysis, the BPN can be viewed as a form of non-parametric multiple regression, but it is free from the assumptions of linearity, normal distribution or regular relationship between measurements. Additionally, trained BPNs are particularly useful as carriers of complex algorithms to transform sets of data from one domain to another.

The SOM consists of neurones arranged in a regular pattern in one or more dimensions, each containing the same number of weights as the expected input data. Input data are matched with every member of the map to find the best fit (winner). The weights of the winner neurone and its neighbours are then adjusted towards the input values, so that they are more likely to become winners when matched with similar patterns. This process is repeated, so that clusters of neurones which are similar to each other but different from those in other clusters in the map appear as demonstrated in Fig. 8.8.

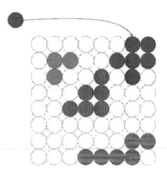

Fig. 8.8. Schematic representation of a self-organising map (SOM) neural network. The different shadings represent clusters or families of neurones that are similar. The number of neurones within a family represents the variation within that family. In a SOM, an input pattern is matched to all neurones in the map; the neurone with the closet matching memorised pattern to the input being the winner.

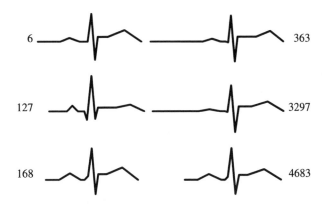

Fig. 8.9. Clustering of fetal electrocardiograms waveforms by a self-organising map neural network into six distinct species or types. The number against each image represents the number of waveforms that are similar in form.

The SOM, therefore, is able to cluster input data according to similarities. Given a sufficiently large map, clustering can be made to any defined level of discrimination and accuracy. It can be viewed as a form of non-parametric cluster analysis, but is free from the assumptions of linearity, normal distribution or regular relationship between measurements. A trained SOM can be used to classify the nature of a dataset, as shown in Fig. 8.9.

Organisation of the Information

A complex sequence of data processing is involved in using the fetal ECG, extending from the acquisition of the stream of voltage signals from the fetus to the production of a clinically meaningful indicator for decision-making. There is a need for a clear and logical organisation of how these processes are to take place. During development, there is a need to minimise the impact of changes in one sub-process on the remainder of the system. During validation, the functions and output from each sub-process may need to be individually reviewed and tested. Even if each sub-process is successfully developed, the effects of how and in what sequence they interact with each other may need to be evaluated and changed.

Object-Orientated Structure of the Data and Algorithm

Object-orientated development divides a major development project into a number of more or less independent modules or objects, and defines the rules or algorithms by which objects interact with each other. Each object can therefore be separately developed and tested, and the manner in which they interact can be separately considered and tested.

An object-orientated development strategy is important. Each component of the system can be developed as an independent object, so that its properties and functions can be independently assessed. This independence also reduces the impact of changes in any component on the remainder of the system. Lastly, the validity and functions of the components can be separately tested from the manner in which the components are arranged in sequence and the rules by which they interact with each other. Development, testing and modifications can therefore take place in a stable and logical environment.

Currently, ECG interpretation systems are developed and presented as a single integrated system, and systems from different developers often behave differently, so standardisation and improvement are not possible. An object-orientated approach allows the sub-processes from different systems to be isolated, so that similarities and differences can be compared. This would make strengths and weaknesses of different applications easier to identify and promote evolution towards better interpretation systems.

The major objects in fetal CTG interpretation are the acquisition and treatment of the electrical signals, the construction of the ECG waveform, the construction of ECG components to indicate fetal response to physiological or pathological events, and the transformation of the physiological information into clinically meaningful indicators.

On the clinical side, similar objects, such as the clinical history, signs and symptoms, and the results of other tests are constructed, leading towards a comprehensive picture of fetal well-being.

The information system for intrapartum decision-making can therefore be viewed as a cluster of interacting objects, demonstrated in Fig. 8.10, while the fetal monitoring object itself is a cluster of objects, as shown in Fig. 8.11. One of the objects in fetal monitoring is the production of a

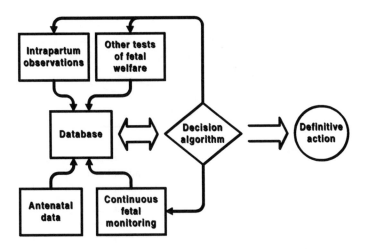

Fig. 8.10. Conceptual representation of an information system for intrapartum decision-making, showing the likely interaction between distinct interacting objects with the system.

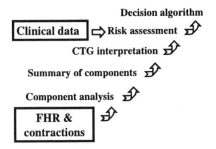

Fig. 8.11. The fetal monitoring component is itself made of hierarchical modules which firstly identify the primary measurements, such as baseline and acceleration. These can then in turn be used to generate summaries of the changes in fetal heart rate for decision-making in other modules and for integration with clinical data.

baseline, itself a further cluster of objects at a lower level, as demonstrated in Fig. 8.12. It can be seen from this approach that the development of the components are quite independent of each other, and changes can be made to a component without severely disrupting the whole system.

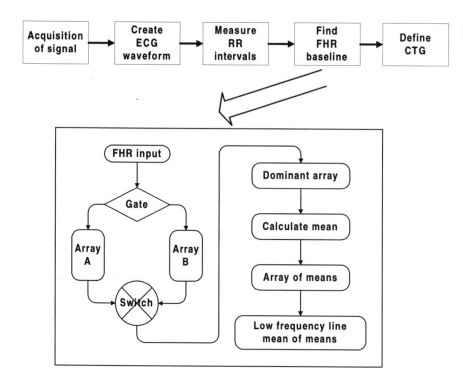

Fig. 8.12. Baseline object deconstructed into its individual subcomponents which produces a low frequency line to represent the baseline.

The arrangement of the objects and the rules by which they interact with each other are equally important, although they do not affect the development of the component objects themselves. An example of how the sequencing of object may affect function is shown in Fig. 8.13. Whether the fetal ECG is used to modify a clinical diagnosis or whether clinical features are used to modify the interpretation of an ECG abnormality, the outcome will result in different decisions in many cases. This is because clinical and ECG abnormalities do not always occur simultaneously.

Object-orientated organisation of information therefore allows a flexible weighting of importance on different components within a system without distorting the components themselves. For example, the information derived

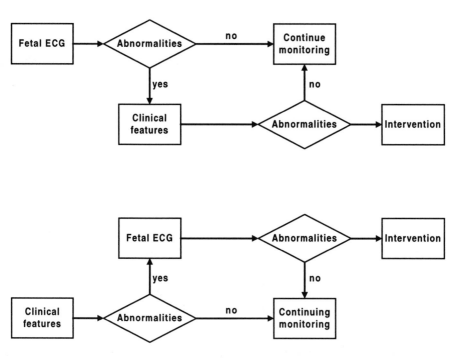

Fig. 8.13. Example of the effect of object sequencing on the decision of whether to intervene or not. The decision will be different depending on which order and at what time the abnormalities are detected and presented.

from the CTG, T/QRS ratio and PR–RR intervals forms individual objects, but the relative importance of these components in deriving a clinical decision can be adjusted according to the user without any change to the three objects.

Presentation

The ability of the computer to present data is well recognised, and currently, this includes the ECG waveform and derivatives of the ECG such as heart rate.

The ability of the computer to present information that is more directly useful for clinical decision-making, however, has not been widely explored. Clinicians vary widely in the manner with which they weigh the importance of input information, and agreements towards a common decision algorithm are difficult to achieve. The medico-legal liability of offering a decision also far exceeds that of accurately reflecting a physiological signal, and this deters the marketing of decision algorithms.

The development of decision support is therefore lacking, and often this consists of a display of alarm to attract attention when physiological measurements exceed a set normal limit, in the form of sound or flashing screen signal. Such displays, however, do not reflect the manner by which clinicians make decisions, which depends on a weighted combination of observations and estimation of risks, and finally choosing a course of action amongst a number of options.

The computer may assist in displaying information through the various stages of decision-making, using the following processes.

Display of normality and abnormality

Physiological signals and observations can be represented as 0 for normal and 1 as abnormal values. Where the observation is a measurement, the logistic transformation results in a number between 0 and 1 representing degrees of abnormality. Multiple measurements can be combined using a neural network or other formulation, so that a low-risk situation can be represented as 0 and high-risk as 1. In this way, a normalised scale can be produced and a uniform method of display can be achieved.

Vector display

Observations and assessment of the fetus are often repeatedly made over a period of time, and risk assessment often depends on the cumulative results of measurements made in the past as well as the most current observations. An example is the measurement of deceleration areas during labour, where both the overall amount of deceleration since labour began

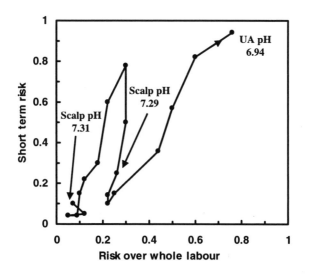

Fig. 8.14. Example of a possible two-dimensional risk-scoring system showing both short-term and whole-labour risk status.

and the current extent of decelerations need to be taken into consideration. A two-dimensional display can be used to display both considerations, as shown in Fig. 8.14.

Chapter 9

CONCLUSIONS

Monitoring Methods Currently in Use

There is an extensive body of literature which is based on fetal monitoring, most of which is based on the use of pulsed Doppler ultrasound and has not therefore been reviewed in this book as we have confined ourselves to work that is based on the use of the R–R′ interval from the fetal ECG.

Measurement and transcription of the R–R′ interval into fetal heart rate is the most accurate way to measure the gross and micro-patterns of the time intervals between successive fetal ECG complexes. Yet, despite the mass of literature that has now been published on the subject, the conclusions are less than satisfactory. There are a number of reasons why the expectations have not been realised.

It has generally been forgotten that the reasons for the development of electronic heart rate monitoring was to prevent unexpected fetal death. It was not introduced to prevent fetal brain damage and, indeed, it has proven to be ineffective in preventing brain damage for a number of reasons. Certainly, there is no evidence that the presence of an abnormal fetal heart rate pattern antenatally does more than reflect damage that has already been inflicted on the fetal brain stem. There is good evidence to suggest that at least 80% of all cases of cortical and brain stem damage are the result of events that precede the onset of labour and are congenital or infective, or due to events that jeopardise placental function. Furthermore, the windows between being alive and normal, alive and abnormal or being dead are quite narrow. If three infants in every thousand can be expected to suffer from cerebral palsy or mental retardation, or indeed a restriction in their developmental potential, then less than 1:1000 is likely to be the result of events during parturition. The introduction of any new method of monitoring and the proof that such a technique has superior sensitivity and specificity over existing methods and will reduce the incidence of brain damage require a very large number of patients if the level of improvement is to achieve statistical significance. Add into this equation errors that may arise in the technology itself, such as signal artefacts or loss of signal strength, and further compound the situation by the well-known vagaries and inconsistencies in the interpretation of CTGs and it can be seen why the introduction of new methods is fraught with difficulties. It can also be seen why conventional fetal heart rate monitoring has fallen into a degree of disrepute with everyone, except lawyers.

Yet, in Europe, North America and Australasia, fetal heart rate monitoring continues to be the proscribed method of intrapartum observation of the fetus and is likely to remain so until some simpler and more robust methodology is developed. The reason for this impasse in technical progression is now particular driven by the law courts, and although large studies may provide the basis of a defence in cases of fetal brain impairment, the fact is that the courts tend to concentrate only on the particular case under review and not unreasonably make the assumption that if a particular method is widely used, then it must represent the current state of the art in management. One of the authors of this book was asked to comment on the following case scenario:

> *A young 16-year-old female was admitted to hospital under the care of a general practitioner obstetrician who was well versed in the current literature on fetal monitoring. The young woman was accompanied by her mother who sat with her throughout labour. The GP examined the woman shortly after her admission. The membranes were intact and contractions were occurring every ten minutes. The cervix was effaced and 3 cm dilated, and the fetal head was engaged in the pelvis. He was asked by the midwives whether they should attach a fetal monitor and he replied in the negative. He was aware that*

large-scale trials had demonstrated no advantages of electronic monitoring over intermittent observations by intermittent auscultation with a fetal stethoscope. He left the hospital.

Labour accelerated and, one hour later, the membranes ruptured spontaneously with the release of meconium-stained amniotic fluid. At the same time, profound fetal bradycardia was observed and the on-call registrar was called. He examined the woman and found the cervix to be fully dilated with the head deeply engaged. He applied forceps and delivered the baby promptly and without any difficulty. The child was profoundly depressed at birth and required active resuscitation. It subsequently showed all the signs of a profound hypoxic ischaemic encephalopathy and went on to be severely spastic and disabled.

In the subsequent legal proceedings, the mother alleged that she had heard the midwives' initial enquiry about monitoring the fetus, which had been denied, and that as a result, the child was now permanently damaged resulting in the impoverishment of both the life of the child and of the mother for the foreseeable future.

No one could in reality be sure that the two events bore any relationship to each other but any competent counsel acting on behalf of the mother would have to ask the obstetrician whether he could be certain — not in the generality of such matters but in this particular case and under these particular circumstances — that the situation would not have been better had he acceded to the original requests of the midwives to apply an electonic fetal heart rate monitor. The case was settled out of court.

In many legal actions for fetal brain damage, the cases are lost because there are long time intervals when the CTG is grossly abnormal and no action is taken. The question must inevitably arise as to why the bother to monitor at all if no action is to be taken, even accepting that abnormalities in the heart rate may be the result of events that have preceded the onset of labour.

There can be little doubt that these uncertainties have resulted in a substantial increase in the Caesarean Section rates and that FHR monitoring is a technique that is highly sensitive but lacks specificity. The need, therefore, is for a more robust and discriminant method by which we can observe the fetus during labour and thereby avoid the need to expedite delivery by operative intervention. There is of course a counter-argument that goes something like this:

> *Most women in more affluent societies now have only one or two children. Vaginal delivery is associated with damage to the pelvic floor resulting in urinary incontinence and often damage to the anal sphincter resulting in incontinence of flatus or feces in a significant number of women. Caesarean Section is a remarkably safe procedure under present-day anaesthesia and surgery. Cerebral palsy and mental retardation are life-long disorders that, in their severest forms, not only disable the child but often completely disrupt the life of the parents, frequently resulting in divorce and great bitterness. Almost inevitably, this type of scenario results in litigation, so why should any woman or her attendants take any risks?*

It is possible that the application of computing methods that recognise patterns of abnormalities of FHR may reduce the vagaries inherent on the clinician's interpretations but using heart rate as a predictor must still provide a very limited window to fetal assessment.

Problems with the Present Systems

The introduction of computer science into the interpretation of the fetal electrocardiogram has made substantial progress. One of the problems is that the systems of FECG analysis produce a vast amount of information about the gross electrical activity in the fetal heart and the interpretation of these data has now reached a high level of sophistication. No doubt the technology will continue to grow as the power of computers grows and their size becomes even smaller. However, much of the progress that has been made in isolating the small repetitive signals from the fetal heart and, in the isolation of these signals from the background electrical noise, has been achieved by creating a running average of the signal. On occasions, this type of technology will fail because the averaging is based around the R wave and therefore fails where there is perseveration between the P wave and the QRS complex.

None of these systems for ECG analysis functions reliably and to their full capacity without a good interface between the subject and the machine and the lowest common denominator is the attachment of the electrode to the presenting part.

Changes based on waveform analysis are more robust when based on time intervals rather than on morphology simply because of the need to use single electrode systems in clinical practice. It may be in the future that the development of procedures that enable reliable collection of data from abdominal electrodes may minimise the effect of electrode placement on the presenting part, and hence, improve the reliability of waveform morphology as a method of fetal monitoring.

The further development of SQUID technology, which in its present form, is expensive and clumsy, may do away with the need to attach any electrodes to the mother or fetus.

Has the Fetal ECG Analysis Enhanced the Specificity of Fetal Monitoring?

Some facets of the FECG waveform are remarkably robust, such as the QRS interval, and only really change in the agonal phases between fetal life and death. Hence, such changes are of little relevance in the management of labour. Furthermore, techniques that use averaging procedures to remove recurrent electrical noise and to enhance the clarity of the signal do occasionally result in the loss of important information. The longer the period of averaging, the more likely it is that detail will be lost. However, with the possible exception of profound periods of fetal bradycardia, major conduction defects are relatively uncommon and errors from short-term averaging do not produce major problems in the assessment of the fetal ECG.

Based on animal data and on human observations, there is good evidence that shifts in the ST segment and the T wave height are associated with hypoxaemia and therefore should be useful in enhancing the specificity of fetal monitoring. Yet, the data from trials on human subjects are conflicting, particularly when viewed in the context of multicentre trials. There are various possible explanations but most of the trials using the T/QRS ratio and PR/FHR ratio have probably made a mistake by including FHR in the ECG arm of their studies.

In a large multicentre trial on the use of the PR/FHR ratio on a short-term and a long-term basis, Strachan *et al.* (2000) performed a retrospective investigation of 679 women in labour. Using a receiver-operator characteristic curve for both T/QRS and PR/FHR ratios, they showed a significant relationship of time interval analysis (PR/FHR) and outcome as judged by the presence of a low umbilical cord arterial pH and base excess at delivery. Such a relationship could not be demonstrated where morphology characteristics (ST segment and T wave height) were used.

However, when a randomised trial using FHR in one arm and FHR + PR/FHR in the other arm was performed by the same group in a large multicentre trial (Strachen *et al.*, 2000), the authors concluded that whilst there was a trend to reduce the operative intervention in the FECG arm, the difference was not significant. There was also no difference in the incidence of unsuspected acidaemia. When Van Wijngaarden *et al.* (personal communication) reanalysed this study, they concluded that only half of the cases in the intervention group showed protocol adherence, and had proper protocol adherence been observed, the figure of intervention would have fallen by 46%. These authors pointed out that protocol adherence was such that cases randomised to both arms of the study were effectively managed by the CTG.

Thus, in multicentre trials for the future, the design should include CTG in one arm and ECG analysis in the other arm if a conclusion is to be reached. The fact is that, despite an enormous amount of work, the question of the value of FECG analysis in clinical practice remains unresolved and is likely to stay unresolved unless investigators are prepared to have a trial that does not include the CTG in both arms. This argument is also likely to be the case with multicentre trials on the T/QRS ratio.

The Way Forward

This is a book about fetal electrocardiography and, therefore, this discussion is not about where we go with fetal monitoring in general but rather it is about where we go with the analysis of the fetal ECG. Because the value of the FECG in labour has not been resolved, there is a need in the future to redesign the structure of the trials, having learnt from previous errors. It may still be that changes in the ECG are too late to provide information in time to prevent damage. In view of the small number of cases where the cause of fetal brain dysfunction is currently believed to be due to events in labour, large trials are required to prove benefit. Benefit is therefore much more likely to be demonstrated in a safe reduction in operative intervention, so this aspect of evaluation still needs to be pursued. However, apart from further improvements in the technology of obtaining and processing the fetal ECG, the interface between clinician and machine needs to be improved. Most governmental equipment agencies are very cautious about the use of systems that make analyses and present judgements to clinicians advising clinical decisions. Yet, provided those observations have been validated and are introduced with appropriate safeguards, there seem to be no reason why progress should not be made in this field. Everyday, large aircraft carrying many hundreds of passengers make landings that are entirely based on computer analysis of complex information. Such methods have been validated and tested for many years. Why not introduce the same principles into fetal monitoring where it is all too evident that we are locked into a technology, which in terms of heart rate, is largely outdated, and where the conservatism of clinicians is reinforced by the demands of the legal system.

Neural networks have been extensively used in the business world but are viewed with some suspicion, as unlike multivariate transformations, it cannot be seen as to how they arrive at their decisions. Self-organising maps enable the clustering of data with similarities but it must also be remembered that the monitoring of fetal welfare consists of a number of interacting objects and objectives, and cannot be reached with the use of the FECG alone.

Finally, the presentation of data by the computer plays an essential role in determining how the clinician will respond and behave. Computer presentations can change dynamically and can switch scaling with the opportunity to move from the particular to the general. Screens can easily be adapted and customised so that clinicians and midwives see only relevant information and are therefore not confused in a way that is currently reflected in the interpretation of CTGs.

REFERENCES

Abboud S & Beker A. *J Electrocardiol* (1989) **22**(Suppl): 238–242

Abboud S & Sadeh D. *J Biomed Eng* (1990) **12**: 161–164

Abduljabbar HS *et al*. *Int J Gynaecol Obstet* (1993) **42**: 251–254

Anonymous. *Am J Obstet Gynecol* (1997) **177**: 1385–1390

Ahlstrom ML & Tompkins WJ. *IEEE Trans Biomed Eng* (1985) **32**: 708–713

Antonucci MC *et al*. *Med Eng Phys* (1997) **19**: 317–326

Arduini D *et al*. *J Perinat Med* (1994) **22**(Suppl 1): 22–27

Attehog JH & Loogna E. *J Electrocardiol* (1977) **10**: 331–336

Barbaro V *et al*. *Med Biol Eng Comput* (1991) **29**: 129–135

Barela TD *et al*. *Clinics Endocrin Metabol* (1983) **12**: 429–446

Beard RW *et al*. *J Obstet Gyneacol Br Commwlth* (1971) **78**: 865–880

Bell GH. *Br J Obstet Gynaecol* (1938) **45**: 214

Bernardes J *et al*. *J Perinat Med* (1991) **19**: 61–65

Bernardes J *et al*. *Int J Gynaecol Obstet* (1998) **62**: 141–147

Bernardes J *et al*. *Br J Obstet Gynaecol* (1996) **103**: 714–715

Bernstine RL *et al*. *Am J Obstet Gynecol* (1968) **101**: 856–857

Bhargava V. *J Electrocardiol* (1994) **27**: 353–255

Blair E & Stanley FJ. *J Pediatrics* (1988) **112**: 515–519

Brambati B & Pardi G. *Br J Obstet Gynaecol* (1980) **87**: 941–948

Brambati B & Pardi G. *Br J Obstet Gynaecol* (1981) **88**: 1233

Bunn AE *et al*. *Med Biol Eng Comput* (1994) **32**(Suppl 4): S58–S59

Caldeyro-Barcia *et al.* (1966) Control of human fetal heart rate in labor. In: (Ed. Cassels ED) *The Heart and Circulation in the Newborn and Infant.* Grune and Stratton, New York, USA, pp. 7–36

Cano GG *et al. J Electrocardiol* (1990) **23**(Suppl): 176–183

Carreti N *et al. Eur J Obstet Gynecol Reprod Biol* (1989) **33**: 281–286

Ceballos-Picot I. (1997) Chapter 2 Biology of oxidative stress. In: *The Role of Oxidative Stress in Neuronal Death.* Chapman Hall, New York, USA

Cheng Q *et al. Comp Biomed Res* (1987) **20**: 428–442

Cerutti S *et al. Clin Phys Physiol Meas* (1989) **10**(Suppl B): 27–31

Chung TK *et al. Br J Obstet Gynaecol* (1995) **102**: 454–460

Cicinelli E *et al. Int J Biomed Comput* (1994) **35**: 193–205

Copel JA *et al. Am J Obstet Gynecol* (1995) **173**: 1384–1390

Copel JA *et al. Obstet Gynecol Clin North Am* (1997) **24**: 201–211

Cremer M. *Muenchener Medizinischen Wochenschrift* (1906) **53**: 811–813

Crowe JA *et al. J Perinat Med* (1996) **24**: 43–53

Dalton KJ *et al. Am J Obstet Gynecol* (1977) **127**: 414

Dalton KJ & Dawson AJ. *Int J Biomed Comput* (1984) **15**: 311–317

Davidsen PC. *Acta Obstet Gynaecol Scand* (1971) **50**: 45–49

Davis J & Meares SD. *Med J Aus* (1954) **2**: 501–504

Dawes NW *et al. Am J Obstet Gynecol* (1999) **180**: 181–187

Dawes GS *et al. J Perinat Med* (1991) **19**: 47–51

De Courten-Myers GM *et al. Biomed Biochem Acta* (1989) **48**: 143–148

De Haan *et al. Am J Obstet Gynecol* (1995) **172**: 35–43

De Haan *et al. Am J Obstet Gynecol* (1996) **174**: 803

De Long ER *et al. Biometrics* (1988) **44**: 837–845

Dennis J *et al. Am J Obstet Gynecol* (1989) **161**: 213–220

Di Renzo GC *et al. J Perinat Med* (1996) **24**: 261–269

Dobbs SE *et al. J Clin Eng* (1984) **9**: 197–212

Donker DK (1991) *Interobserver Variation in the Assessment of Fetal Heart Rate Recordings.* Academic Proefschrift VU University Press, Amsterdam.

Dressler M & Moskokowitz SN. *Am J Obstet Gynec* (1941) **41**: 775

Easby MH. *Am Heart J* (1934) **10**: 118–119

Edington PT *et al. BMJ* (1975) **1**: 7–9

Escalona OJ *et al. Med Biol Eng Comput* (1993) **31**(Suppl): S137–S146

Family JM. (1982) Cross correlation techniques applied to the fetal electrocardiogram. PhD thesis, University of Nottingham

Favret AG. *Med Biol Eng* (1968) **6**: 467–475

Fawthorp DJ *et al. Arch Toxicol* (1991) **65**: 437–444

Fee SC *et al. Am J Obstet Gynecol* (1990) **162**: 802–806

Ferarra ER & Widrow B. *IEEE Trans Biomed Eng* (1982) **29**: 458–460

Ferrazzi E *et al. Clin Phys Physiol Meas* (1989) **10**(Suppl B): 57–60

FIGO. *Int J Gynaecol Obstet* (1987) **25**: 159–167

Forbes AD & Jimison HB. *J Clin Monit* (1987) **3**: 53–63

Friesen GM *et al. IEEE Trans Biomed Eng* (1990) **37**: 85–98

Gardosi J. (1995) *2nd ISIS Symposium*, Dublin

Genevier ES *et al. Med Eng Phys* (1995) **17**: 514–522

Gennser G & Nilsson E. *Acta Physiol Scand* (1968) **73**: 42–53

Gelli MG & Gyulai F. *Acta Obstet Gynaecol Scand* (1969) **48**: 56–63

Gibson NM *et al. Med Eng Phys* (1995) **17**: 188–196

Gilstrap LC *et al. Am J Obstet Gynecol* (1989) **161**: 825–830

Greene KR. *Curr Opin Obstet Gynecol* (1996) **8**: 123–127

Goldaber KG *et al. Obstet Gynecol* (1991) **78**: 1103–1107

Goodwin TM *et al. Am J Obstet Gynecol* (1992) **167**: 1506–1512

Groome LJ *et al. Early Hum Dev* (1994) **38**: 1–9

Guid Oei S *et al. BMJ* (1989) **298**: 568

Gulmezoglu AM *et al. Br J Obstet Gynaecol* (1996) **103**: 513–517

Guzman ER *et al. J Matern Fetal Med* (1998) **7**: 43–47

Greene KR *et al. Am J Obstet Gynecol* (1982) **144**: 950–958

Gross KR *et al. Clin Exper Rheumatol* (1989) **7**: 651–657

Haesslein HC & Niswander KR. *Am J Obstet Gynecol* (1980) **137**: 245–253

Hammacher K. Hewlett Packard editions No. 5953 (1978) 1109

Hanley JA & McNeil BJ. *Radiology* (1982) **143**: 29–36

Haverkamp AD *et al*. *Am J Obstet Gynecol* (1979) **134**: 399–408

Heard JD *et al*. *Am Heart J* (1936) **11**: 41–48

Helliwell B & Gutteridge JMC. *Lancet* (1984) **8391**: 1396–1397

Hioki T. *Acta Obstet Gynaecol Jap* (1975) **22**: 162

Hofmeyr GJ *et al*. *Br J Obstet Gynaecol* (1993) **100**: 649–652

Hokegard KH *et al*. *Br J Obstet Gynaecol* (1978) **85**: 165–170

Hokegard KH *et al*. *Acta Physiol Scand* (1981) **113**: 1–7

Hon EH. *Am J Obstet Gynecol* (1963) **91**: 772–774

Hon EH. (1968) *An Atlas of Fetal Heart Rate Patterns.* Harty Press Inc., New Haven, Connecticut, USA

Hon EH & Hess OW. *Science* (1957) **125**: 553–554

Hon EH & Huang HS. *Obstet Gynecol* (1962) **20**: 81

Hon EH & Lee ST. *Med Arts Sci* (1963) **15**: 120

Hon EH & Lee ST. *Obst Gynecol* (1964) **24**: 6

Hon EH & Lee ST. *Am J Obstet Gynecol* (1963) **87**: 804

Hon EH & Lee ST. *Am J Obstet Gynecol* (1963) **87**: 1086–1096

Hon EH & Lee ST. *Am J Obstet Gynecol* (1965) **91**: 59–60

Hynal C & Kellner DZ. *Klin Med* (1924) **98**: 365

Ikenoue T *et al*. *Am J Obstet Gynecol* (1981) **141**: 797

Ingemarrson I *et al*. (1993) *Fetal Heart Rate Monitoring.* Oxford University Press, p. 54

Ingemarrson I *et al*. (1993) *Fetal Heart Rate Monitoring.* Oxford University Press, p. 113

Jenkins HML *et al*. *Br J Obstet Gynaecol* (1986) **93**: 6–12

Kadambe S *et al*. *IEEE Trans Biomed Eng* (1999) **46**: 838–848

Kahn AR. *Proceedings of the 16th Annual Conference on Engineering in Medicine and Biology* (1963) **5**: 134

Kaplan S & Toyama S. *Obstet Gynecol* (1958) **11**: 391–397

Karin J *et al*. *Pediatr Res* (1993) **34**: 134–138

Katz M *et al*. *Obstet Gynecol* (1979) **54**: 372–374

Kaneoka T *et al*. *Surg Forum* (1961) **12**: 421–422

Keith RD *et al*. *Br J Obstet Gynaecol* (1995) **102**: 688–700

Keith RD *et al*. *Med Biol Eng Comput* (1994) **32**(Suppl 4): S51–S57

Kendall B *et al*. *Am J Obstet Gynecol* (1964) **90**: 340

Kennedy E. (1833) *Observations on Obstetric Auscultation: An Analysis of the Evidences of Pregnancy*. Hodges and Smith, Dublin

Knopf K *et al*. *J Dev Physiol* (1991) **16**: 367–372

Kohonen T. (1984) *Self Organization and Associative Memory*, 2nd edn. Springer-Verlag, Berlin

Komaromy *et al*. *Br J Obstet Gynaecol* (1977) **84**: 492–496

Koster JF *et al*. *Life Chem Rep* (1986) **3**: 323–325

Krebs HB *et al*. *Am J Obstet Gynecol* (1943) **145**: 297–305

Kubo T *et al*. *Am J Perinatol* (1987) **4**: 179–186

Kwon J & Shandas R. *Biomed Sci Instrum* (1996) **32**: 87–92

Lamkee MJ *et al*. *Am J Obstet Gynecol* (1962) **83**: 1622

Larks SD. *Am J Obstet Gynecol* (1959) **77**: 1109–1115

Larks SD. *Am J Obstet Gynecol* (1965) **91**: 46

Larks SD & Anderson GV. *Am J Obstet Gynecol* (1962) **84**: 1893

Larks SD & Larks GG. *Am J Obstet Gynecol* (1966) **15**: 553–555

Larks SD & Larks GG. *Biol Neonat* (1966) **10**: 140–152

Larks SD & Larks GG. *Am J Obstet Gynecol* (1995) **93**: 975–983

Larks SD & Longo L. *Obstet Gynecol* (1962) **19**: 740

Lee KH & Blackwell RJ. *Obstets Gynaecol Brit Commwlth* (1974) **81**: 61–69

Lee ST & Hon EH. *Obstet Gynecol* (1963) **22**: 553

Levine S. *Am J Path* (1960) **36**: 1–17

Ligtenberg A & Kunt M. *Comp Biomed Res* (1983) **16**: 273–286

Lindecrantz KG & Lilja H. *J Biomed Eng* (1988) **10**: 280

Lindecrantz KG *et al*. *J Biomed Eng* (1988) **10**: 351–353

Lindecrantz KG *et al*. *Int J Biomed Comput* (1993) **33**: 199–207

Lilja H *et al*. *Br J Obstet Gynaecol* (1985) **92**: 611–617

Lilja H *et al*. *Int J Gynaecol Obstet* (1989) **30**: 109–116

Lotgering FK *et al*. *Am J Obstet Gynecol* (1982) **144**: 701–705

Low JA *et al. Am J Obstet Gynecol* (1988) **158**: 356–361

Low JA *et al. Am J Obstet Gynecol* (1990) **163**: 1131–1135

Low JA *et al. Am J Obstet Gynecol* (1994) **170**: 1081–1087

MacDonald *et al. Am J Obstets Gynecol* (1985) **152**: 524–539

MacLachlan NA *et al. Br J Obstet Gynaecol* (1992) **99**: 26–31

Maeda K. *Baillieres Clin Obstet Gynaecol* (1990) **4**: 797–813

Maekawa M & Toyoshima J. *Acta Sco Med Univ Imp Kioto* (1944) **12**: 519

Mann H & Bernstein P. *Am Heart J* (1941) **22**: 390–400

Mantel R *et al. Int J Biomed Comput* (1990) **25**: 261–272

Mantel R *et al. Int J Biomed Comput* (1990) **25**: 273–286

Maragnes P *et al. Pediatrie* (1991) **46**: 481–488

Marvell CJ & Kirk DL. *J Biomed Eng* (1980) **2**: 216–220

Mazzeo JR. *Med Prog Technol* (1994) **20**: 75–79

McLennon A *et al. BMJ* (1999) **319**: 1054–1059

Mohajer MP *et al. Eur J Obstet Gynecol Repr Biol* (1994) **55**: 63–70

Mohajer MP *et al. Arch Dis Childhood* (1995) **72**: F51–F53

Mongelli M *et al. Br J Obstet Gynaecol* (1997) **104**: 771–774

Mongelli M *et al. Br J Obstet Gynaecol* (1997) **104**: 1128–1133

Mongelli JM *et al. Acta Obstet Gynecol Scand* (1997) **76**: 765–768

Morgan M & Symonds EM. *Eur J Obstet Gynecol Reprod Biol* (1991) **42**: 9–13

Muller-Schmid P. *Geburtsh Frauenheilk* (1959) **19**: 401

Murphy KW *et al. Br J Obstet Gynecol* (1992) **99**: 32–37

Murray HG. *J Perinatal Med* (1986) **14**: 399–404

Murray HG. (1992) Evaluation of the fetal electrocardiogram. MD thesis, University of Nottingham.

Myers RE. *Am J Obstet Gynecol* (1972) **112**: 246–276

Myers RE *et al. Am J Obstet Gynecol* (1973) **115**: 1083–1094

Natale R *et al. Am J Obstet Gynecol* (1988) **158**: 317–321

Newbold S *et al. Br J Obstet Gynaecol* (1991) **98**: 173–178

Newbold S *et al. J Obstet Gynaecol* (1989) **96**: 144–150

Nielsen PV *et al. Acta Obstet Gynecol Scand* (1987) **66**: 421–424

Okada M. *IEEE Trans on Biomed Eng* (1979) **26**: 700–703

Pardi G *et al. Amer J Obstets Gynecol* (1974) **118**: 243–250

Pardi G *et al.* (1971) Electrocardiographic patterns and cardiovascular performance of the sheep fetus during hypoxia. In (Eds. Crosignani PG & Pardi G) *Fetal Evaluation During Pregnancy and Labour*. Academic Press, London, pp. 157–174

Pardi G *et al. Contr Gynec Obstet* (1977) **3**: 22

Pardi G *et al. Br J Obstet Gynaecol* (1986) **93**: 250–254

Parer JT & Livingston EG. *Am J Obstet Gynecol* (1990) **162**: 1421–1427

Park YC *et al. IEEE Trans Biomed Eng* (1992) **39**: 868–871

Pello LC *et al. Obstet Gynecol* (1991) **78**: 602–610

Pharoah P *et al. Arch Dis Childhood* (1996) **75**: F169–F173

Phoenix RG *et al. Med Prog Technol* (1993) **19**: 89–103

Pinsky WW *et al. Clin Obstet Gynecol* (1991) **34**: 304–309

Quinn A *et al. Br J Obstet Gynaecol* (1994) **101**: 866–870

Raichle ME. *Ann Neurol* (1983) **13**: 210–217

Reed NN *et al. Eur J Obstet Gynecol Repr Biol* (1996) **68**: 87–92

Rhyne, VT. *Amer J Obstet Gynecol* (1968) **102**: 549–555

Rhyne, VT. *Med Res Eng* (1970) **9**: 8–10

Roche JB & Hon EH. *Am J Obstet Gynecol* (1965) **92**: 1149–1159

Roemer *et al.* (1972) *Proceedings of the International Symposium on the Treatment of Foetal Risks*, Baden, Austria, pp. 135–159

Rogers MS *et al. Gynecol Obstet Invest* (1997) **44**: 229–233

Rogers MS *et al.* (1997) *4th ISIS Symposium, Paris*

Rogers MS *et al. Br J Obstet Gynaecol* (1998) **105**: 739–744

Rosen KG *et al. Acta Physiol Scand* (1976) **98**: 275–284

Rosen KG & Isaksson O. *Biol Neonate* (1976) **30**: 17–24

Rosen KG & Kjellmer I. *Acta Physiol Scand* (1975) **93**: 59–66

Rosen KG & Westgate J. *Am J Obstet Gynecol* (1996) **174**: 802

Rumulhart DE *et al.* (1986) Learning internal representation by error propagation. In (Eds. Rumelhart DE, McClelland JL & PDP Research Group) *Parallel Distributed Processing Explorations in the Microstructure of Cognition Volume 2: Foundations*. The MIT Press, Cambridge, MA, pp. 318–362

Sachs H. *Pfuegers Arch* (1922) **197**: 536

Saugstad OD. *Paediatr* (1996) **98**: 103–107

Schneider H *et al.* *Obstet Gynecol* (1977) **50**(Suppl 1): S58–S61

Scott DE. *Med Res Eng* (1970) **9**: 7

Seitz I. (1903) Die fetalen Herztone unter der geburt Munchen Habil-Schrift

Shenker L. *Obstet Gynecologic Rev* (1966) **21**: 367–388

Shield JEA & Kirk DL. *J Biomed Eng* (1981) 44–48

Shields JR & Schifrin BS. *Obstet Gynecol* (1988) **71**: 899–905

Sholtz WJ. *Neuropath Exper Neurol* (1953) **12**: 249–261

Shono H *et al.* *Early Hum Dev* (1991) **27**: 111–117

Sibony O *et al.* *Eur J Obstet Gynecol Reprod Biol* (1994) **54**: 103–108

Skillern L *et al.* *Br J Obstet Gynaecol* (1994) **95**: 582–586

Smith PR. (1983) An advanced fetal monitoring system. PhD thesis, University of Nottingham

Smith PR & Kirk DL. *J Perinat Med* (1986) **14**: 391–397

Smyth CN. *Lancet* (1953) **1**: 1124–1126

Socol ML *et al.* *Am J Obstet Gynecol* (1994) **170**: 991

Southern EM. *Am J Obstet Gynecol* (1957) **73**: 233–247

Spencer JAD & Samson I. *Br J Obstet Gynaecol* (1998) **105**(Suppl 17): 83

Steer P. *Br J Obstet Gynaecol* (1982) **89**: 690–693

Steinberg CA *et al.* *IEEE Trans Biomed Electron* (1962) **9**: 22–30

Strassman EO & Mussey RD. *Am J Obstet Gynecol* (1938) **36**: 986–997

Sugarman RG *et al.* *Obstet Gynecol* (1978) **52**: 301–307

Supnet MC *et al.* *Pediatr Res* (1994) **36**: 283–287

Sureau C. *Gynec Obstet* (1956) **55**: 521–533

Symonds EM. *J Obstet Gynaecol Br Commwlth* (1971) **78**: 957–970

Symonds EM. *J Obstet Gynaecol Br Commwlth* (1972) **79**: 416–423

Symonds EM. *Aust NZ J Obstet Gynaecol* (1972) **12**: 170–175

Thaler I *et al.* *J Perinat Med* (1988) **16**: 373–379

Tipton RH & Shelley T. *J Obstet Gynaecol Br Commwlth* (1971) **78**: 702–706

Todros T *et al.* *Eur J Obstet Gynecol Repr Biol* (1996) **68**: 83–86

Tompkins WJ & Pan J. *IEEE Frans Biomed Eng* (1985) **32**: 230–235

Unger FW & Goodwin JW. *Am J Obstet Gynecol* (1972) **112**: 351–357

van Wijngaarden WJ *et al. Am J Obstet Gynecol* (1996) **174**: 1295–1299

van Wijngaarden WJ *et al. Am J Obstet Gynecol* (1996) **175**: 548–554

van Woerden *et al. J Perinat Med* (1991) **19**: 73–80

van Woerden EE *et al. Int J Biomed Comput* (1990) **25**: 253–260

Vara P & Niemineva K. *Acta Obstet Gynecol Scand* (1951) **132**: 241

Vindla S *et al. Fetal Diagn Ther* (1997) **12**(6): 319–327

Wade ME *et al. Obstet Gynecol* (1976) **48**: 287

Wakai RT *et al. Early Hum Dev* (1993) **35**: 15–24

Wang CC & Rogers MS. *Br J Obstet Gynaecol* (1997) **104**: 251–255

Wang W *et al. Am J Obstet Gynecol* (1996) **174**: 62–65

Ward RJ & Peters TJ. (1995) Free radicals. In *Clinical Biochemistry: Metabolic and Clinical Aspects* (Eds. Marshall WJ & Bangert SK) Churchill Livingstone, New York, pp. 765–777

Webster JG *et al. Med Biol Eng Comput* (1983) **21**: 343–350

Weiner CP & Thompson MI. *Am J Obstet Gynecol* (1988) **158**: 570–573

Westgate J *et al. Clin Phys Physiol Meas* (1990) **11**: 297–306

Westgate J *et al. Lancet* (1992) **340**: 194–198

Westgate J *et al. Ped Res* (1998) **44**: 297–303

Whitfield CR. *Am J Obstet Gynecol* (1966) **95**: 669–675

Widmark C *et al. J Dev Physiol* (1992) **18**: 99–103

Widrow *et al. Proc IEEE* (1975) **63**: 1692–1716

Wilcox MA *et al. Obstet Gynecol* (1997) **89**: 577–580

Winckel F. (1893) Lehrbuch der Geburtshilfe einschliesslich der Pathologie und Therapie des Wochenbetts. Fur praktische Aerzte und Studirende 2 Aufl Leipzig, Veit & Co

Winkler CL *et al. Am J Obstet Gynecol* (1991) **164**: 637–641

Xue Q *et al. IEEE Trans Biomed Eng* (1992) **39**: 317–329

Yeh MH *et al. Am J Obstet Gynecol* (1975) **121**: 951–957

Youden WJ. *Cancer* (1950) **3**: 32–35

Young BK *et al. Obstet Gynecol* (1979) **54**: 427–432

Index

abdominal electrodes   2, 9, 27
abdominal leads   2
abdomino-rectal leads   2
abnormal auto-antibodies   112
abnormal heart rate patterns   32
absent FHR variability   74
absent P wave   11
absent variability   72
accelerations   74, 75, 80, 120
accumulation of waste products   32
acid–base   14
acidosis   23
acidotic infant   16
acquisition   53
action potential   90
active electrode   54
actocardiogram   30
acute fetal compromise   98
acute hypoxia   32
acutely asphyxiated fetal lambs   95
adaptive algorithm   122
adaptive noise cancelling   63
adenosine diphosphate (ADP)   33
adenosine transport inhibitor   106
adenosine triphosphate (ATP)   33, 104
adrenaline infusion   12
algorithms   58
amiodarone   113
amplitude   104
amplitude measurements   65
anaerobic glycolytic pathway   34
analogue-to-digital converter   63
analysis   30
anencephalic fetus   8
animal model   47
antenatal fetal heart rate   30
antepartum accelerations   74
antepartum fetal heart rate   81
anti-La and anti-Ro   112

antibodies   112
antioxidants   37
aortic arch   35
aortic stenosis   23
Apgar score   14
apoptosis   38
area   92
arrhythmias   20
assessment of variability   86
atrial bigeminy   24
atrial fibrillation   115, 116
atrial flutter   115
atrial myocardial cells   51
atrial myocardium   50
atrial trigeminy   110
atrioventricular block   10
atrioventricular (A/V) node   50, 70
atrioventricular conduction system   92
atrioventricular heart block   11
atrium   70
auricular fibrillation   24
automaticity   50
autonomic nervous system   71
autoregulation   71
AV node(s)   70, 96
averaging techniques   11
axis measurements   102

back propagation neural network   87
back-propagation network (BPN)   123
balanced input amplifier   2
balloon probe   55
band pass filters   59
bandwidth   8
baroreceptor reflex   75
baroreceptors   70
basal heart rate   70
base changes   10
baseline   79, 83, 120

baseline drift   63
baseline fetal heart rate   71
baseline tachycardia   76
baseline variability   29, 30, 74, 75, 79
baseline wander   106
basic processing unit   122
Baysean probability analysis   121
biophysics   49
biphasic   11
biphasic T waves   8
bipolar electrode arrangement   57
bipolar scalp electrode   57
birth weight   20, 21, 102
blocked atrial premature beats   111, 112
bradycardia(s)   5, 111
breech presentation   3
bundle of His   50

calcium channel blocker   106
cardiac arrhythmias   23, 108
cardiac axis in early labour   22
cardiac axis shift   102
cardiac catheterisation electrode   5
cardiac failure   114
cardiac response   32, 35
cardiotocography   99, 101
cardiotocography plus PR   101
carotid baroreceptors   70
carotid bodies   35
carotid sinus   70
"CAT" (computer of averaged
    transients)   60
CAT computer   6
catecholamine(s)   51, 70
catecholamine surges   16
cellular damage   32, 38
cerebral blood flow   xi
cerebral palsy   ix, x, 77
changes in rate   3
changing PR/FHR relationship   96
chaos   87
chemoreceptors   35, 70
chronically   95
chronically instrumented lambs   12

clinical trial of predictive tests   46
cluster analysis   122
coherent averaging   27
common decision algorithm   130
common iliac compression   97
complete atrioventricular heart block   24
complete heart block   70, 111–113
computerised algorithms   79
computerised assessment   78
computerised estimation   83, 84
computerised identification   87
computerised systems   30, 81, 83
conduction index   16, 17, 96–100
conduction of the impulse   22
congenital heart disease   23, 115
congenital mitral   23
congestive cardiac failure   116
congestive heart failure   116
Copeland clip   54, 56
Copeland electrode   56
Copeland scalp electrode   55
cord artery pH   16
cord blood acid–base measurements   9
cord lactate   16
cord occlusion   97
cord venous blood   13
cord venous blood lactate   12
corrected QT   10
creatinine phosphate   12, 104
CTG   120, 129
CTG versus CTG + CI   17
cytochrome reactions   33
cytochrome system   34

death   114
DEC LSI-11/23 computer   13
deceleration(s)   74, 80, 87, 88, 120, 121
decision logic   58
decision-making   127
declining membrane potential   97
dehydrogenase   33
dehydrogenase reactions   33
delayed decelerations   2
depletion   12

depolarisation   51, 90
depression   5, 8, 11
dexamethasone   113
dichotomisation of heart rate   119
digital converter   63
digital high-pass filter   85
digoxin   114, 116
direct intrauterine electrode   5
discriminant analysis   121
distortion   63
DNA damage   38
Doppler ultrasound   26, 29, 71
double-spiral   54
drugs   74
Dublin randomised study   ix
duration   93
Dutch system   81
dying fetus   8

early decelerations   75, 80
ECG parameters   16
ECG waveform(s)   59, 117
"éctopic" beats   109
EFM versus EFM + FECG   100
"Einthovens Triangle"   53
electrical activation   52
electrical activation in the heart   50
electrical axis   21, 22
electrical axis vector   22
electrode characteristics   56
elevation   9, 10, 13
encephalopathy   38
enhanced running-averaged waveform   60
enhanced waveform   64
enhancement   58
enlarged P waves   7
epinephrine   70
escape rhythms   108, 111
excessive baseline drift   64
excessive maternal caffeine intake   110
external electrodes to the abdomen   3
extrasystoles   23, 108, 109

false negatives   41
false positives   41

fast Fourier transformation   120
fast oxygen   90
FECG baseline   6
FECG parameters   99
female fetuses   95
fetal acidosis   x, 30
fetal baboons   10, 92
fetal behavioural states   73
fetal blood gas and pH   34
fetal bradycardia   18, 137
fetal brain damage   132, 134
fetal cardiac   22
fetal cardiac arrhythmias   23, 108
fetal condition at birth   99
fetal conduction system   112
fetal distress   2, 31
fetal electrocardiogram   49, 52, 89
fetal growth retardation   20
fetal heart   36, 70
fetal heart rate   ix, 29, 30, 74
fetal heart rate regulation   69
fetal hypoxaemia   17, 75
fetal hypoxia   7
fetal lambs   12, 92
fetal malformations   74
fetal myocardial conduction system   95
fetal myocardium   xi
fetal physiological response to
    hypoxia   33
fetal QRS complex   18
fetal radio-electrocardiography   9
fetal scalp blood pH   15
fetal tachycardia   10
fetal vector cardiography   102
FHR variability   73, 74
fibrillation   109
FIGO definition   30
FIGO guidelines   79
8–50 Hz filter   6, 8
flecainide   113, 115, 116
flutter or paroxysmal tachycardias   24
fractals   87
fraying of the genetic strands   38
free fatty acids   34
free hydroxyl radicals   36

free-oxygen radicals   xi
free radicals   37
frequency characteristics   56
frequency determination   87

Gardosi and Spencer probes   56
general anaesthesia   74
genetic   x
glycogen   12, 104
good frequency response   90
Göteborg   11
Göteborg system   14
group-averaging technique   60
growth retardation   21

Hammacher's classification   72
hardware amplifiers   63
Hawthorne effect   46, 47
heart block   112
heart rate   13
heart rate baseline   120
heart rate changes   36
heart rate variability   70
height of the T wave   67
high altitude   22
high fetal heart rate variability   73
high frequency component   85
high plasma potassium   10
high signal amplitude   90
high-pass filter(s)   3, 9
high-pass filtering   3
hydrogen   33
hydrops   113
hyperkalaemia   23
hyperstimulation of uterine activity   103
hypoxaemia   93, 96, 137
hypoxanthine   16, 36, 99
hypoxia   74, 103, 104
hypoxia in primates   73
hypoxic damage   32

immune heart block   112
increased variability   72

"indifferent" electrode   54
induced asphyxia   12
inefficient action   113
influx of Ca^{++} 90
initial embryological appearance   69
input weightings   124
insensitive Na^+ 90
intermediary metabolism   33
intermittent auscultation   ix, 5
interobserver agreement   78
interobserver variability   30
interpretation of CTGs   133
intervals   89
intervention and morbidity   46
intervention benefit ratio (IBR)   42, 46
intervention rates   99
intra-observer variabilities   78
intracellular potassium loss   10
intrapartum asphyxia   77
intrapartum decision-making   127
intrapartum fetal heart rate   83
intrapartum fetal hypoxia   39
intrauterine silver wire   4
intraventricular conduction time   21
intraventricular conduction time of fetal
    heart   20
inversion   9, 11, 93
inverted P wave   7
inverted T waves   5, 8
ischaemia   xi
isoelectric line   13
iterative approximation   124

K^+ ion efflux   97
ketoacids   34
ketone bodies   34
Kohonen   123

lactacidosis   12
lactate levels   104
lactate values in cord arterial samples   14
lactic acid   34
large multicentre randomised trial   101

late decelerations   11, 75, 76, 80
late labour   22
lead II QRS   22
left-axis shift   22
lengthening   9
lidocaine   116
linear filter   58
line-fit routine   91
lipoproteins   37
log noradrenaline   16
$\log_{10}$ norepinephrine   99
long-term fetal heart rate variability   85
long-term increase   104
long-term variability   71, 72, 87
longer time interval   21
low birth weight infants   ix
low fetal heart rate variability   73
low signal-to-noise ratio   90
low variability   74
low-pass digital recursive filter   60

major conduction defects   137
male   95
male and female infants   21
male infants   21
management criteria   100
matching algorithms   58
maternal aortic compression   10
mature infants   ix
mean electrical axis   103
medulla oblongata   69
metabolic acidosis   12, 34
microfluctuation   71
mild late decelerations   92
morphology   64, 89
multilead system   27
multiple regression analysis   121
multiple sensors   55
multivariate transformations   120
myocardial contractility   36
myocardial hypoxia   12
myocardial mass   102

myocardium   12

Na^+ ion influx   97
NADH   33
National Institute of Child Health
  (NICH)   79
necrotising enterocolitis   38
negative diagnostic value (NDV)   42
negative PR/FHR   96
negative waveform   3
neural network functions   123
neural networks   xii, 59, 122, 123, 139
neuronal processing units   123
neurone   122
nicotinamide adenine dinucleotide (NAD)
  33
nodal tachycardia   26, 114
noise reduction   6
non-immune hydrops   112
non-linear transformation   58
non-parametric cluster analysis   125
non-parametric multiple regression   124
non-penetrating electrodes   54
noradrenaline levels   13
norepinephrine   70
normal variability   72
notching   19, 93
Nottingham   11
Nottingham fetal ECG analyser   100
Nottingham system   81, 91, 93

object sequencing   129
object-orientated development   126
object-orientated organisation   128
object-orientated structure   126
observational studies   101
optimal placement   3
oronasal cavity   22
oscillations   72
Oxford Sonicaid System 8000   81
oxygen radical(s)   36, 38
oxygen saturation   5, 35

oxygen tension   10

P wave   4, 12, 49, 52, 93, 136
P wave area   93
P wave duration   13
P wave morphology   92
P–R interval   117
pacemaker   50, 70
pacemaker cells   90, 97
pacemaker sites   50
parasympathetic activity   70, 72
parasympathetic fibres   70
parasympathetic (vagal) nerves   50
parasympathetic nervous system   71
parasympathetic regulation   74
parasympathetic response   36
parturition   x
patterns of heart rate   30
period of tachycardia   121
permanent neurological deficits   32
phonocardiography   3, 29
plastic probe   55
Plymouth trial, 1993   104
PORTO system   81
positive diagnostic value (PDV)   42
positive waveform   3
power spectral analysis   59
power spectrum   87
PQ   9
PQ interval(s)   5, 10, 92
PR   9, 13
PR & FHR   16
PR interval(s)   4, 5, 7, 10, 12, 13, 91, 95
PR segment   67
PR/FHR   95, 137
PR/FHR correlation   95
PR/FHR ratio(s)   101, 137
PR/FHR relationship   93
PR–RR   129
PR/RR relationship   97
pre-term hydropic fetus   114
prediction   99
predictive capacity   99
predictor and outcome variables   121

pregnant monkeys   10
prevalence   ix
pro-arrhythmic effects   115
probes   54
problem-solving methods   123
problem-solving techniques   122
procainamide   116
profound fetal bradycardia   23
prolongation   10
prolonged PR interval   5
prolonged QT interval   11
prolonged SVT   114
propanolol   116
prospective randomised trial   101
protocol adherence   137
pulsed Doppler ultrasound   72, 132
Purkinje fibres   50

Q wave   52
QRS   64
QRS complex   4, 8, 18, 49, 52, 102, 104, 136
QRS detectors   58, 59
QRS duration(s)   5, 18–21, 26, 102
QRS interval   136
QRS waveform   58
QRS width   26, 102
QT interval   9, 10, 103

R wave   19, 52
R wave height   95
R wave in the fetal ECG   29
R–R' duration   103
R–R' interval   29, 69, 132
R/S ratio   22, 102
R/S relationship   102
radicals   xi
randomised controlled trials   45
randomised study   17, 100
randomised trial   16
ratio index   16, 17, 97, 98, 99, 100
real time analysis   13
receiver operating curve (ROC)   44

receiver operational characteristics
   (ROC)   43
receiver-operator characteristic curve   137
reduced variability   72, 74
regulatory impact   71
relationship   13, 16, 102
respiratory acidaemia   93
retrograde atrial activation   116
rhesus iso-immunisation   72
right-axis shift   22
rocainamide   116
RR   13
RR interval   78
running-weighted-averaging
   techniques   60

S wave   52
S–T segment changes   6
SA   70
SA node   93, 96
saltatory pattern   73
sampling interval   86
scalp blood   9, 15
scalp clip   6
scalp electrodes   9, 53, 56
second-order low-pass Butterworth
   recursive digital filter   62
self-organising map (SOM)   123, 139
self-organising map (SOM) neural
   network   124
sensitivity   41
serial transformation   120
severe fetal anaemia   72
sheep studies   106
short-chain ketoacids   34
short-term variability   72, 87
signal   53
signal artefacts   133
signal detection   58
signal distortion   2
signal isolation   11
signal-to-noise ratio(s)   6, 19
"silent" flat trace   72
silent pattern   72
simple transformations   117

single hollow ventricle   69
single spiral electrodes   90
single-use probes   55
sino-atrial (SA) node   50, 70, 90
sinus arrhythmia   3
sinus bradycardia   111
sinusoidal patterns   72
slow Ca^{++} 90
slow oxygen-dependent channel   93
specific auto-antibodies   112
specificity   41
Spencer electrode   56
Spencer probe   55
spiral electrode   54, 56
spirals   56
splitting   19
spring-loaded clip   54
ST segment   xii, 5, 8–13, 95, 103, 104,
   137
ST segment analyser (STAN)   14, 16
ST segment changes   12
ST segment depression   9, 11
ST waveform   104
ST waveform analysis   15
stainless steel pincer electrode   54
Stan system   67, 106
statistical evaluation of continuous
   predictors   43
statistical evaluation of discrete
   predictors   41
straight-line model   67
superconducting quantum interference
   device (SQUID) technology   27, 136
supraventricular extrasystoles   23, 109
supraventricular rhythms   108
supraventricular tachycardia(s)   113
sympathetic activation   74
sympathetic nerves   50
sympathetic response   35
syntactical algorithms   58
systemic lupus erythematosis   112

T wave   4, 8, 9, 11, 12, 49, 104
T wave amplitude   11, 12
T wave configuration   xii, 12, 103

T wave elevation   10
T wave height   10, 12, 13, 103, 104, 137
T wave inversion   11
T/QRS   12, 14, 15, 104, 105, 129, 137
T/QRS ratio(s)   12–14, 67, 101, 104, 105
T/QRS value   12
tachyarrhythmia(s)   24, 26
tachycardias   109, 133
taxonomy   121
theoretical assumptions   118
thresholding algorithms   58
time-coherent enhanced averaging
    (TCEA)   60, 63, 91
time intervals   65
time-coherent filtering process   13
toxins   32
transformations   118
transient noise spikes,   63
trigeminal rhythm   23
trigeminy   24
true negatives   41
true positives   41
two-dimensional risk-scoring system   131
type 2 dips   75
typical variable decelerations   76

umbilical artery pH   15
umbilical cord   22
unbilical arterial blood   5
umbilical venous blood   5
umbilical venous noradrenaline   93
unipolar lead configuration   57
uric acid   36
uterine activity   102
uterine contractions   30

vagal and vasomotor centres   70

vagal stimulation   92
vagal tone   70
vaginal electrode   53
vaginal leads   4
validation of predictive tests   44
value in the neonate   22
valve amplifier   2
variability   36, 71, 84, 120
variable decelerations   10, 76, 80
vector analysis   102
vector display   130
vector-cardiography   8
vectors   57, 102
ventricular arrhythmias   24
ventricular extrasystole(s)   109, 110
ventricular myocardial cells   51
ventricular myocardium   50
ventricular predominance   22
ventricular tachycardia   116
vertex presentation   3
vibro-acoustic stimulation   73, 75

wandering pacemaker   19, 26, 114
wave height   117
waveform   63
wavelet transformations   59
weight differences   95
weighted running average   91
weighted-averaging technique   60
widened QRS complex(es)   5, 19
width of the QRS   102
Wolff–Parkinson–White syndrome   114

Youden index   42, 43

Z transform   118
Z-transformed product   98

DEMCO